MEN AND BOOKS

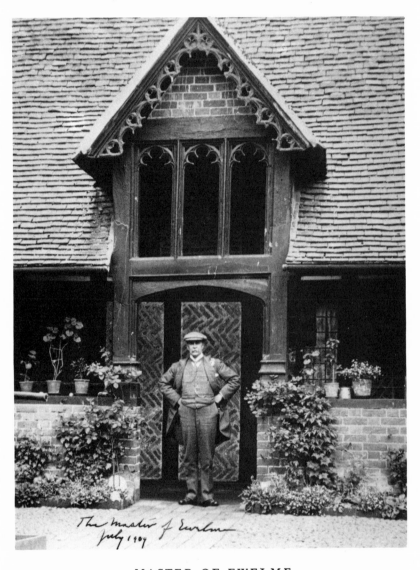

MASTER OF EWELME

As Regius Professor of Medicine at Oxford Osler was, by tradition, Master of the Almshouse of Ewelme, residence of thirteen aged Almsmen. This photograph was made by Dr. George Dock three years before the Men and Books articles were begun.

MEN
AND
BOOKS

BY SIR WILLIAM OSLER

Collected and reprinted
from the
Canadian Medical Association Journal
With an Introduction by

EARL F. NATION, M.D.

THE SACRUM PRESS

Durham, North Carolina

1987

THE SACRUM PRESS

8 CHANCERY PLACE

DURHAM, NORTH CAROLINA 27707

ISBN 0-937543-01-2

DEDICATED BY THE EDITOR

TO THE MEMORY

OF

GEORGE DOCK

AND BY THE PUBLISHER

TO THE MEMORY

OF

WILLIAM WILLOUGHBY FRANCIS

Contents

INTRODUCTORY NOTE

THE *"Men and Books* snippets" as Osler was wont to call the pieces collected here, were begun in 1912 when the author, then Regius Professor of Medicine at Oxford, was 62 years of age. They were written in response to the request for some "thunder" by his friend, the new editor of the *Canadian Medical Association Journal,* Dr. Andrew McPhail. They appeared fairly regularly during the years 1912, 1913, and 1914. They ceased when Osler became too involved in the strife and turmoil of the war.

With his Canadian background, Osler had a warm feeling for the Canadian Medical Association and for his friends who were responsible for it. It was not without some sentiment, therefore, that he was willing to see his work buried in the Association's new journal. However, as a consequence, most Osler followers have seen only fragments of these articles which were published in twenty-six installments.

Osler had a high reverence for great men of the past and great books were his lifelong passion. This veneration seemed to furnish him with an inexhaustible supply of material for such articles as these. The pieces are interesting, enjoyable, and instructive. It therefore seems worthwhile to collect them within a single cover that they may be more accessible.

In addition to being delightful accounts of men and books, these vignettes reflect much of the character and humanity of the beloved physician, teacher, and scholar who wrote them. Perhaps they will give pleasure and inspiration to others as they have to me.

EARL F. NATION, M.D.

PASADENA, 1959

I. *Nicolaus Steno*

THE Danes have good reason to be proud of the series of distinguished men who have graced the profession of that country in the past three hundred years. No one should have a warmer place in our memory than the anatomist, geologist, and theologian whose name is on our lips daily in connexion with the duct of the parotid gland. There has recently been published in Copenhagen at the expense of the Carlsbergfond [an institution corresponding to one of the Carnegie Foundations], and edited by Vilhelm Maar, *Nicolai Stenonsis Opera Philosophica,* in two sumptuous volumes. The edition is limited, but it should be in the hands of all important medical libraries. It may be obtained from Vilhelm Tryde, Copenhagen, and the price is 50 kroner.

An excellent introduction, in English, gives an account of Steno's life and work. After studying with the famous Bartholins, father and son, he went to Amsterdam, where in his twenty-second year he made the discovery with which his name is associated. Then he studied with the famous Sylvius, of Leyden, and after a disappointing visit to his native city, where he had hoped to obtain a professorship, he went to Paris and then to Florence. In addition to anatomical studies, he seems to have everywhere taken a great interest in religious conditions, and in Florence he was gradually won over to Catholicism. By this time he had done a great deal of good anatomical work on the lymphatic vessels, the brain, the heart, and the muscles, and also in comparative anatomy, and the papers are reproduced in these volumes.

The very day he renounced his Protestant faith Steno was summoned to the University of Copenhagen by the Danish king, but he did not take up his work there as Anatomicus Regius until 1672, and he found the conditions so unfavourable that he resigned after two years.

The scientific work of Steno is more appreciated to-day in geology than in anatomy. During his prolonged visits in Florence

1

he became interested in the geological conditions of Tuscany, and his studies in palaeontology were among the first to determine the exact nature of fossils. He also made important generalizations on stratification. A few years ago the International Society of Geologists erected a tablet to his memory in the court of the Laurentian library at Florence.

From brilliant studies in science Steno was early diverted to religious problems, and in 1675 he took orders in the Roman Catholic Church and devoted the rest of his life to the service of God and the church. With a singular charm of manner and great personal piety he was soon surrounded in Florence by hosts of friends, and so much was he appreciated that in 1677 he was appointed Bishop of Titiopolis "in partibus infidelium," and Vicar Apostolic of Northern Germany and Scandinavia. For a time he lived in Hanover, then in Münster, and lastly in Hamburg. He sold all his property and lived the life of an ascetic, and made long, troublesome journeys. At Hamburg the austerity of his life became so extreme that he did nothing to live up to his rank, did not even wear his clerical suit, and spent everything on the poor. So ardently did he work for the church that he made himself hated even by the Catholics, who threatened to cut off his ears and drive him from the town as a criminal. In 1685 he left Hamburg for Schwerin, "where he worked under circumstances which were, if possible, still more distressing, and here he died in unspeakable misery, forty-eight years old." The Grand Duke of Tuscany had his body removed to Florence, where it rests in the crypt of St. Lorenzo. A strange figure, one of the strangest in our history, well worthy of the affectionate tribute which his countrymen have paid in these two splendid volumes.

II. *Les Collections Artistiques de la Faculté de Médecine de Paris*

THERE may be faculties with finer buildings, there are some with better laboratories, but there is none of any country with such a history, or with such treasures, artistic and literary, as the medical faculty of Paris. And this is as it should be, since in time it outdates all but Oxford and Bologna, and in long centuries of importance it out-classes all others. The most cherished possession of its magnificent library, second only to that of the Surgeon-General's in Washington, are the twenty-five manuscript volumes of *Commentaries* from 1395 to 1786—incomparable annals, as Corlieu says, written by the hands of the one hundred and ninety-four deans who successfully became heads of the school, and who related in these volumes the important acts of their administrations. And there were earlier records, but Dr. Hahn, the learned librarian of the faculty, told me he did not think there was medical instruction before 1200, and that the date of the first doctorate was 1270.

But the object of this note is to call attention to a sumptuous work in large quarto issued by Masson et Cie (100 francs), and edited by Noé Legrand, Dr. Hahn's able coadjutor in the library, and published under the care of the present dean, Professor Landouzy.

After a description of the buildings and pictures of the present faculty, and their gradual evolution, there follows a set of beautiful reproductions of the portraits in the possession of the faculty, many of great artistic, and all of historical, importance. There are fine early pictures of Guy De Chauliac; Pitard, the great thirteenth century surgeon; and many of the men who in the fifteenth and sixteenth centuries made Paris famous, Fernel, Piètre,and Riolan. One above all others is interesting to the historical student, Gui Patin (1601-1672), author of the famous letters which give such

3

a life-like picture of the medical profession in France in the seventeenth century. Legrand quotes a happy description of him by Vigneul-Marville: "Il était satirique depuis la tête jusqu'aux pieds. Son chapeau, son collet, son manteau, son pourpoint, ses chausses, ses bottines, tout cela faisait nargue à la mode et le préces à la vanité. Il avait dans le visage l'air de Ciceron, et dans l'esprit le caractère de Rabelais. Sa grand mémoire lui fournissait toujours de quoi parler, et il parlait beaucoup. Il était hardi, témeraire, inconsidère, mais simple et naïf dans ses expressions. Il s'exprimait en latin d'une manière si recherchée et si extraordinaire que tout Paris accourait à ses theses comme à une comédie."

Then follows a group of about fifty portraits of the celebrated members of the College and Academy of Surgery; afterwards the portraits of the modern men who have made the school since the fusion of the College of Surgery with the old faculty. There are splendid pictures of Laennec, of Nélaton, and of Trousseau. The faculty is very rich in sculptures, of which there are reproductions of more than one hundred.

Among the most treasured possessions of the medical school are the famous Gobelin tapestries, executed in 1634. They are in a splendid state of preservation, and are beautifully reproduced in this volume. Then follows a description of the various designs, engravings, medals, and the different works of art in the possession of the faculty. It is a magnificent volume, full of historical interest, and exposes for the first time to full light the wonderful treasures of the Paris school.

4

III. *Samuel Wilks*

WHEN a student in Montreal, during the summer of 1871, I had an opportunity to make a good many post mortems at the General Hospital, and with the material so collected I wrote my graduation thesis. It was my habit to pester Dr. Palmer Howard for information and literature, and one day he handed to me Wilks's *Lectures on Morbid Anatomy,* and from that time everything was plain sailing, as all the ordinary appearances met with were described fully. This was my first introduction to the well-known Guy's Hospital physician. When a student in London, Mr. Arthur Durham, one of the surgeons at Guy's, whom I knew quite well, took me to Dr. Wilks's wards one day, and I have very pleasant recollections of a delightful visit.

In 1875 I sent him a copy of a study which I had made of a remarkable case of a miner's lung, which I had obtained from the body of a Novia Scotian miner who had died under my care in the small-pox department of the General Hospital, and to this day I can recall the great pleasure I felt at the kindly letter I received in acknowledgment, the first of a great many which he wrote to me, always in the same sympathetic way. I did not meet him socially until 1878, when I was in London with Dr. George Ross. I sent our cards in one day as he was "making the rounds" at Guy's. I was surprised that he left the bedside group with such rapidity after receiving our cards, but he rushed up to us and with some embarrassment, and with his eyes twitching, asked "For Heaven's sake, do either of you speak French?" He was struggling with an exceedingly inquisitive professor from Bordeaux, and fortunately Dr. Ross was able to act as intermediary. We spent a delightful evening at his house, and thereafter it was my habit, on visits to London, always to call upon him.

Few men in the profession had a longer or better innings. With his death snaps the last link between the old medicine and the new, the link which united the profession with the famous clinicians of

5

the early part of the last century, Bright, Addison, and Hodgkin. Wilks may be said to have stood sponsor to both Addison and Hodgkin, and his best work was probably in helping to clearly define the diseases described by them. He illustrated the advantages and disadvantages of approaching clinical medicine through the dead house. Knowing disease thoroughly, he became a great diagnostician, but his training fostered the therapeutic nihilism into which he, Gull, and many of his contemporaries were driven, and for which, when we think of the vagaries of those days, we have to be greatly thankful. He was a frank, outspoken man, whose yea was yea, and nay, nay, to students and patients alike.

Wilks's life may be read in his recently issued *Biographical Reminiscences,* which gives a charming picture of his early years, and of the Guy's Hospital School, of which he was in our generation the chief ornament. While not a great autobiography, like that of Kussmaul, it has the merit of a well-told story, without needless padding, and rich in details of a period memorable in our history. He had a remarkably attractive personality, which age so adorned, that at three score and ten there was no handsomer man in London. A good head, well-moulded features, merry blue eyes, and abundant white hair made up an ideal picture. And he had all the things that should accompany old age: fairly good health to the end, an unceasing interest in life, and the affectionate esteem of a large circle of friends.

The last time I saw him in public was at Guy's Hospital, about five years ago, when I gave an address on Sir Thomas Browne. He was then over eighty, and had recently recovered from an appendicitis operation. It was delightful to see the just pride which the Guy's students took in the dear old man, to whom they listened with eager attention. Blest with the saving salt of humour, he reminded one sometimes of the Autocrat of the Breakfast Table, to whose works he was devoted. In their outlook on life they had much in common, as Holmes himself remarked in a charming letter which is given in Morse's life. Wilks had a delicious honesty which sometimes bordered on the indiscreet, and which did not always make his advice as a consultant acceptable. And on the occasions at which it was his duty to read biographical notices, the "verum" rather than the "bonum" was emphasized. But these traits only added to the charm of a great physician and an honest man.

6

IV. *Jean Astruc*
and the Higher Criticism

IT IS strange how the memory of a man may float to posterity on what he would have himself regarded as the most trifling of his works. Ask in succession a score of doctors, "Who was Astruc?" and the expression aroused indicates that at least in our profession he is "clean forgotten as the dead man out of mind"; and yet librarians and dealers in second-hand books know only too well what a prolific writer he was in the first half of the eighteenth century. But ask any theologian, any man interested in the history of the Bible, the same question, and his face at once brightens—or darkens—as he replies, "Oh, Jean Astruc, he was the father of modern biblical criticism." And so it is that the man whom we have forgotten, who cut such a figure in the profession at Montpelier and Paris, the enumeration of whose tomes extends through three pages in the *Biographie Médicale,* is remembered today by a small octavo volume, published anonymously in Brussels, 1753, with the title, "Conjectures sur les Mémoires Originaux dont il paroit que Moyse s'est servi pour composer le Liver de la Genese. Avec des Remarques, que appuient ou qui éclaircissent ces Conjectures."

Interested in Astruc for some years, having had occasion to refer to his splendid work on the history of syphilis and to his history of the Montpellier faculty, and incidentally knowing his position as the founder of the criticism of the Pentateuch, I had long tried to get the above named volume, which I had never seen advertised in any catalogue. It turned up the other day at Sotheby's in the Huth collection. I sent a bid to Quaritch with the admonition "not to lose it"; and as the book is of great rarity I expected to pay a reasonably high price; but, illustrating the hazard of the auction room, no one seemed to know of it and it fell to me for a few shillings.

The story of Astruc's medical life is fully given in Bayle's *Biographie Médicale.* His position in modern theology may be gleaned from an eight-page article in the recent *Real Encyklopädie für Protestantische Theologie.* In Genkel's Encyklopädie, Baentsch says, "from the appearance of this book dates the fruitful

7

criticism of the Pentateuch. That in the following century its problems have been solved is owing to Astruc, the significance of whose work is assured for all time. The year 1753 in which the book appeared is a milestone in the history of the science of the Old Testament."

Though published in 1753, it was composed some time previously, but the author hesitated to publish lest "les prétendus esprits forts" should regard it as lowering the authority of the Pentateuch; but a learned and religious friend overcame his scruples, urging that the arrangement of Genesis in parallel columns according to its sources would be no greater change than was its division into chapters and verses.

Of the two ways by which Moses could have had his information, oral tradition, "de bouche en bouche," or by written documents which had been handed down, the first was regarded as most probable; but in spite of the fewness of lives, owing to the longevity before the Flood, which lent weight to this view, Astruc believed there were insuperable objections to it. A study of the documents forced the conclusion that Moses had access to many ancient documents describing the world since creation, coming from different sources and varying in detail. He patched them together one after another, thus forming the book of Genesis as we have it. Only in this way could the repetitions and contradictions be explained. But Astruc's notable discovery was the recognition that in Genesis there are two separate accounts of the Creation and of the early days of the world, the one extending as far as verse 3 of Chapter II, in which the Creator is spoken of as Elohim, the other extending from verse 4 of Chapter II to the end of Chapter IV, in which the Creator is called Jehovah. These accounts differ in important details, particularly in the fact that in the Javistic account no mention is made of the sin of Adam, which plays so important a rôle in Pauline Christianity. Astruc recognized other sources, and prints in parallel columns under A, B, C, D, the four most important, which he had worked out as far as to the end of Chapter II of the Book of Exodus.

The work is a small octavo volume, extending to 525 pages, fully one-half of which is taken up with a critical consideration of his views. Small wonder that in 1753 the distinguished physician to the king, and professor in the Paris faculty, published such a work anonymously, and in Brussels.

8

v. *Two Frenchmen on Laughter*

LIKE song that sweetens toil, laughter brightens the road of life, and to be born with a sense of the comic is a precious heritage. So much do we differ in the possession of this faculty, that a twentieth-century explanation would seek for differences in quantity or quality of some internal secretion which stimulates the phrenic centres. Or one may prefer the view of Aristotle, who describes the diaphragm (phrenes) as a membrane which when overheated by tickling, so "disturbs mental action as to occasion movements that are independent of the will." In any case, the close connexion believed to exist between the mind and the diaphragm is still suggested to us by the anatomical term "phrenic nerves." We owe to Aristotle the first study of the physiology of laughter, and the recognition of it as a faculty peculiar to man.

Having always held with that philosopher who regarded a day wasted in which he had not had a good laugh, I eagerly read Bergson's *Laughter, an Essay on the Meaning of the Comic* (Macmillan and Co.). What a delightful gift to be able to make smooth the rough places of psychology! With not a dry page, full of thought so clearly expressed and so happily illustrated, and not too long, the book is a model of clear presentation. And yet, to take the end first, philosopher like, he reaches a lame and impotent conclusion at which my Democritean soul rebels; for the final comparison of laughter is with the froth of which a child picks up on a sandy beach a handful, sparkling like gaiety itself, but to the taste the substance scanty and the after taste bitter!

Indifference, absence of feeling, Bergson says, is the natural environment of laughter, which always has a social signification. The trivial mishap that raises a laugh is associated with a mechanical inelasticity—a lack, through failure of mind or of muscle, of adaptability, and the living pliability of a human being. The eccentric in action, at whom we laugh, lacks in character that tension and elasticity which social life brings into play, and upon which its

9

success depends. "The rigidity is the comic and laughter is its corrective." And it is the same with gestures, attitudes and movements of the body, which are comic "in exact proportion as the body reminds us of a machine." So too, the ludicrous in words comes out when an absent idea is fitted into a well-established phrase, as when a lazy lout says, "I don't like working between meals," which has nothing amusing in itself, but only in connexion with the commonplace phrase, "one should not eat between meals."

Protecting itself by laughter, society demands that each member shall be attentive to his social surroundings—he must fit himself to the environment. A comic in character is one who "automatically goes about his own way without troubling to get himself in touch with the rest of his fellows, and it is by laughter we reprove his absent-mindedness and waken him out of his dreams." These hurriedly noted points, taken almost at random, may serve to indicate the rich treat in store for any one who wishes to follow the workings of one of the ablest minds of our generation. The title suggests *Punch* or *Life* in the hands of a vivisector, but instead we find humanity in the retort of a chemist of the soul, and the analysis is presented in formulae of easy comprehension by the plain man.

How scanty the literature on laughter is shown by a glance at the index catalogue of the Surgeon-General's Library. Excluding a few theses and, in series II, reference to papers on spasmodic or uncontrollable laughter, there is mention of three or four monographs, one of which is the only elaborate treatise ever written on the subject—*Traité du Ris,* by M. Laur. Joubert, Paris, 1579—a work noted by Brunet as "recherché à cause du Dialogue sur la Cacographie." Such a contrast to Bergson! We are in another world, with other thoughts, strange terms, and an anatomy and physiology still dominated by Galen. A treatise weighty with authorities, and interspersed with illustrations drawn from Hebrew, Arabic, Greek, and Latin authors, it has, as Brunet remarks, a curious value, apart from the subject-matter, as Joubert was one of the earliest advocates of phonetic spelling, in which style the work is printed, and there is an appendix, "Dialogue sur la Cacographie Françaize." Laughter is discussed in three sections, in the first of which the material is analyzed, and it is interesting to find the same basic elements as given by Bergson: absence of feeling and some mishap or unseemliness—"laideur et faute de pitié"—as when an old fellow plays in the street like a child, or when a gaily dressed beau tumbles in the mud.

There are many shrewd comments on the comic in words and in situations. He has great difficulty in placing the risible faculty, but after a long disquisition on the brain and mind it is finally localized in the heart itself. The mind first perceives the ridiculous and it is communicated at once to the heart by the nerves, as by vessels —"the swift thought," in Shelley's phrase, "winging itself to laughter." The intimate relation of the diaphragm with the heart explains why this structure is the organ of laughter, and one reason why man alone among animals possesses this faculty is the wide extent of the attachment of the human pericardium to the diaphragm.

Various chapters treat the movements of the face and mouth, the scintillation of the eyes, the tears, the redness of the face, the shaking of the shoulders and of the body, the pain in the abdomen and the loss of sphincter control. In the second book he considers the definitions given by authors, and the different species of laughter, and the reasons why men laugh when the diaphragm is wounded. His own definition may be quoted, and it illustrates the phonetic spelling. "Le Ris et un mouvement, fait de l'esprit épandu, et inegale agitacion du coeur qui épanit la bouche ou les laivres, secoüant le diaphragme et les parties pectirales, avec impetuosité et son autrerompu par lequel et exprimée une affeccion de chose laide, indigne de pitié." Whether man is the only creature which laughs, on the men who have neither wept nor laughed, on the influence of the spleen, why one melancholic laughs and another cries, whether a baby smiles before the fortieth day, why great laughers grow fat, on those who have died laughing—are among the subjects considered in Book III.

Joubert, who lived in the palmy days of the Montpellier school and succeeded his old teacher, the famous Rondelet, wrote many works, among which the most celebrated were the treatises on gun-shot wounds and on vulgar errors. From the latter it is not unlikely Sir Thomas Browne had the suggestion for his work on the same subject.

I cavilled at Bergson's conclusion,—that like sea-froth the substance of laughter is scanty and the after taste bitter. It is not always so. Joubert is right. There is a form that springs from the

11

heart, heard every day in the merry voice of childhood, the expression of a laughter-loving spirit that defies analysis by the philosopher, which has nothing rigid or mechanical in it, and is totally without social significance. Bubbling spontaneously from the artless heart of child or man, without egoism and full of feeling, laughter is the music of life. After his magical survey of the world in the *Anatomy of Melancholy,* Burton could not well decide, *fleat Heraclitus an rideat Democritus,* whether to weep with the one or laugh with the other, and at the end of the day this is often the mental attitude of the doctor; but once with ears attuned to the music of which I speak, he is ever on the side of the great Abderite, and there is the happy possibility that, like Lionel in, I think, one of Shelley's poems, he may keep himself young with laughter.

VI. *An Incident in the Life of Harvey*

IT IS remarkable how few letters remain of the great Harvey—
two or three at the British Museum, not many more at the College
of Physicians, one or two at the Bodleian, only a scanty fragment
of what must have been an enormous correspondence throughout
his long and active life. There are some precious Harvey MSS., the
most remarkable of which are the actual notes of his lectures at
the Royal College of Physicians beginning in April, 1616, and
including the very one in which, on April 17th, he demonstrates
for the first time the circulation of the blood. This manuscript was
reproduced in 1886 by a Committee of the College of Physicians
(Prelectiones Anatomiae Universalis).

Notes of his lectures on the muscles still exist in the British Museum, and it to be hoped that they may be published before long.
A great difficulty is in deciphering the atrocious handwriting, and
this may be one of the chief reasons, as Dr. Norman Moore suggests, why so few of his letters survive. It was not worth keeping
letters one could not read!

Recently there has come to light an interesting collection of
about a dozen letters, written in 1636, dealing with an unknown
incident in Harvey's life, when he accompanied the mission of
Lord Arundel to the Imperial Court of Germany. They have been
published by the Historical Manuscripts Commission (Report on
the MSS. of the Earl of Denbigh, 1911). Some details of this
journey we already know, particularly the vain attempt to demon-
strate at Nürnberg to Caspar Hofmann the circulation of the
blood. The letters are addressed to Lord Fielding, who at the time
was ambassador to Venice. He describes the desolate country
through which they had to pass before arriving at Lintz, where
they had their first audience with the Emperor, and where some of
them "went-a-hounting" with him. Then they went to Vienna and
Baden, Prague, and Ratisbon. From the latter place he arranged
to visit his friend the ambassador at Venice, and eight or nine of

13

the letters are concerned with the troubles and difficulties experienced on the journey.

All went well until he reached Treviso, the quarantine station. In spite of his pass, the recommendations from the English king, from the German emperor, and from Lord Arundel, the authorities insisted that his passport was not in proper form, and that he had come from places infected with the plague. Harvey is reputed to have been very quick-tempered, and it must have been terribly trying to him to be detained in a wretched, dirty lazaretto for two weeks, writing frantic letters every day to Lord Fielding imploring the intervention of the government, and of the college at Venice. He slept at first in the open field, as they wished to put him in the lazaretto where he might, as he says, have taken the infection.

The phraseology and spelling of the letters are interesting, *e.g.* "I am a little jealous of them, and to take anny beds now of ther sending, for since ther manners and cruelty hath beene soe shamefull to me, and they have soe little reason for what they have done, it would be like the rest of ther proceedings yf they sent me an infected bed to make ther conjectures and suspitions prove true; therfor I choose to ley still to be redeemed by your Excellency oute of this inocent straw. Yesterday likewise the patron that owed the howse wheare I first took my straw bed (a little poore garden howse full of lumber, durt and knatts, without window or dore, open to the high way att midnight) was to offer me that agayne, because I had chosen that to shun the infamy of this lazeret and the suspition I had that sum infected person had lately bene heare, and from which they forced me with terror of muskets, I write this to shew your Eccellency that all they doe heare upon your stirring is butt formal to salve their own errors."

At last he was released and joined his friend at Venice. After remaining for a time with the ambassador, he went on to Florence and Rome. It is a great pity that we have no letters giving his impressions of the changes at his old school, Padua, where he was a student for so long, but it is interesting to get even this brief glimpse of the great physiologist, though under circumstances so aggravating to him.

14

VII. *Letters of Laennec*

I do not collect autograph letters, but everything relating to Laennec is of such intense interest to me that it was impossible to resist sending a bid at the Van der Corput sale last year at Amsterdam; and I was fortunate enough to secure two letters and a manuscript of the great founder of modern clinical medicine. Laennec MSS. are not numerous. A few years ago I was interested in looking over those which are in the library of the Faculty of Medicine at Paris (No. 399-400 in the catalogue). The most important, notes of lectures on pathological anatomy, have been edited by Cornil (Paris, 1884). There are lecture notes also of his course at the Collège de France in 1822, 1824, and 1825, and also many memoranda relating to cases. There is a rough pencil drawing of an abdominal tumour; post-mortem notes; quotations from Boerhaave, Baglivi, Morgagni, and Sydenham, many of them on little cards 2 x 1½ inches. Baglivi seems to have been a favourite author, as there are a number of slips and extracts from his writings. Among the MSS. there is an interesting and, so far as I know, unpublished discourse on his admission to the Anatomical Society, 1808, in which he speaks of the advantages of the study of pathological anatomy. In it he refers to a usage of the Society, that all communications should be made *de vive voix*—a good rule, still, I am afraid, much honoured in the breach.

There are also incomplete papers on "Blood-clots in the Vessels During Life," "Cartilaginous Bodies in the Joints," and "On Accidental Tissues."

Of the letters which I was fortunate enough to get, one is a very brief note to an astronomer friend, dated 1810, handing on a letter which he had just received from Baltimore describing an unusual astronomical phenomenon. The other, which is dated 1824, is a letter of introduction given to Dr. Villemoneise, who had worked with him at the Necker Hospital. The third MS. is a rough draft of four pages of the obituary notice (written May 12th, 1816) of

15

one of the most lovable of men—Gaspard Laurent Bayle.* Laennec's senior by seven years, Bayle was a man of extraordinary capacity, with, as Chomel remarks in his notice of him, "un esprit infatigable." Not one of the group of distinguished pupils of Corvisart had made such an impression on his contemporaries. He had devoted himself to the subject of tuberculosis, on which his monograph (1810) is still one of the landmarks in our knowledge of the disease. He died of an affection of the chest, probably tuberculosis, at the early age of forty-two, deeply lamented. Laennec concludes his sketch with the words: "Les pauvres regretteront longtemps en lui le médicin qui, en leur donnant ses conseils ne les laissa jamais dans l'impuissance de les suivre; ses confrères, l'homme modeste qui jeune encore était déjà une des lumières de la médicine française; et ses amis, un ami d'un commerce sûr, d'une sagesse profonde, d'une douceur et d'une égalité de caractère à l'épreuve de tous les évenemens."

*His biography in Bayle, *Biographie Medicale,* is well worth reading.

VIII. *Dr. Payne's Library*

THE working library of a doctor is not, as a rule, worth much after his death; but when a man is interested in books, knows their value, and buys judiciously, the collection which he leaves may form a considerable part of his estate. I know an old doctor living not far from here whose hobby for forty years has been first editions, some half a dozen of which are worth his entire establishment.

A scholar and a book lover of the best type, Dr. Joseph Frank Payne began to collect early, and had wide interests, both professional and literary. There was no one in England better versed in the history of medicine, to which he had made a number of contributions of the first rank, principally on Anglo-Saxon medicine. Shortly before his death he delivered in Oxford a most instructive course of lectures on Greek pre-Hippocratic medicine, which it is to be hoped he has left in a state for publication.

Part of his library was sold in July, and the remainder at the end of January. The first portion consisted of between two thousand and three thousand volumes, including many splendid incunabula, a number of choice MSS., ten or twelve old diplomas, many medical portraits, a special collection of works on the plague, and an extraordinary collection of nearly fifteen hundred medical tracts, chiefly English. I was anxious that the library should be kept together, and my friend, Mr. A. W. Marburg of Baltimore, very kindly commissioned me to buy it for the Johns Hopkins Medical School, for which a few years ago he bought a valuable collection of old books. The executors had placed a reserve price of £2,700, but on the morning of the sale I received an intimation that it would be reduced to £2,500. The collection was to be offered first *en bloc*. With Dr. Henry Barton Jacobs and Dr. George Dock, I went to Sotheby's at one o'clock on January 12th. A more rapid sale I never saw. The bidding began at £2,000, and within a minute it was knocked down to an unknown bidder at £2,300, a

17

figure beyond that which Mr. Marburg had mentioned, but Dr. Jacobs and I were prepared to go to the reserve price, had we had a chance! The name of the purchaser is not known, but I believe the collection remains in this country.

The second part of the library consisted of a special collection of about one hundred and sixteen Herbals, a few miscellaneous classical works and a collection of first and other editions of Milton and Miltoniana. The Herbals were offered *en bloc,* but the reserve price was not reached. Several of the fifteenth century Herbals brought a very good price; a 1488 Herbarium, the earliest with figures of plants, brought £96. For years Dr. Payne had been very much interested in Milton, and his collection contained a very large number of first editions. The highest price paid for a single item was for a quarto edition of the famous tract on *Education,* one of the very few copies known in this form, for which Mr. Quaritch paid £172. The library realized as a whole £4,353, a figure which is rarely reached by modern medical collections.

IX. *The Funeral of Lord Lister*

I HAVE just come from the Abbey service—the most splendid tribute ever paid to our profession, and so richly deserved in the person of Joseph Lister, one of the greatest benefactors of humanity. Voltaire saw Newton buried like a king in the same Abbey, and ever after esteemed it one of the glories of England that she was able to recognize the supreme merits of a king among men. Today's ceremony was England's tribute of heart and head. The nation's Valhalla was packed to the doors; nurses, students, doctors, and the general public crowded in the nave, while the reserved seats of choir and transepts were thronged with a gathering of representatives from all parts of Europe.

As one of the delegates from the University of Oxford I had a choir seat, which chanced to be next to our own Chancellor, Lord Strathcona. The recognition of the international character of Lord Lister's work was witnessed by the presence of nearly all the foreign ambassadors, and representatives of the Académies des Sciences of Russia, Sweden and Norway, Spain, and Rome. Among those who occupied seats were the Prime Minister, and many of his colleagues, Lord Lansdowne and the Duke of Northumberland. Opposite to me was a group of Lister's old Glasgow and Edinburgh pupils—MacEwen, Caird, Littlejohn, Bramwell, Balfour, Playfair, and others.

Just before 2.30 p.m., after the organist had finished playing Chopin's "Funeral March," there was heard at intervals a distant voice, high above the silence. At first the impression was of some one singing outside. I was waiting for it, having had a few years ago, at the funeral of Lord Kelvin, the same experience. The choir coming through the cloisters sang the hymn, "Brief Life is here our Portion," and the high note at the end of the third line alone reached us in the clear, liquid voice of one boy. For three or four verses this was heard without another note of the full choir (the sound of which was not audible until the last verse), which fin-

19

ished just as the procession entered the Abbey. Preceded by the canons, the coffin was borne through the nave and choir covered with a purple pall and on it a magnificent wreath of orchids sent by the German Emperor. The pall-bearers were Lord Rayleigh, Lord Rosebery, Lord Iveagh, president of the Lister Institute, the president of the Royal Society, the principal of Glasgow University, the president of the Royal College of Surgeons (Mr. Godlees, Lord Lister's nephew), Sir Watson Cheyne, and Professor Caird. Immediately following the family was a group of foreign delegates, MM. Chauveau, Dastre, and Pozzi from Paris; Garré, president of the German Congress of Surgeons, and Treub from Holland. Professor Chauveau, who must now be the *doyen* of French science, was a very striking figure with his fine face and head, and long white hair. It was a noble and ever-to-be-remembered occasion. And was ever Handel's grand anthem sung more fittingly?

"When the ear heard him, then it blessed him; and when the eye saw him, it gave witness of him. He delivered the poor that cried; the fatherless and him that had none to help him. Kindness, meekness, and comfort were in his tongue. If there was any virtue and if there was any praise, he thought on those things. His body is buried in peace, but his name liveth evermore."

Only those who have lived in the pre-Listerian days can appreciate the revolution which has taken place in surgery. In the seventies at the old Montreal General Hospital we passed through it, and it is pleasant to recall that when Dr. Roddick returned from Lister with the technique there was no opposition, but the surgeons patiently practised a laborious and unnecessary ritual for the sake of the better results. As with everything that is worth preserving in this life there has been evolution, but from the great underlying principle on which Lister acted there has been no departure.

I wonder how many surgeons have taken the trouble to work through the literature of the growth of the method as given in Lister's writings? It is now available, and no surgeon's library is complete without these splendid volumes, published a few years ago by the Oxford Press—a worthy monument for the greatest Englishman of his generation.

20

x. *Gui Patin*

ONE physician we know thoroughly, and one only—Gui Patin, Dean of the Faculty of Medicine, Paris. His ways and works, his inmost thoughts, his children, his wife, his mother-in-law (!), his friends, his enemies—*the latter very well*—his books and pictures, his likes and dislikes, joys and sorrows, all the details of a long and busy life, are disclosed in a series of unique letters written to his intimates between 1630 and 1672. But this is not a biographical note—I wish only to lodge a protest and to express a hope.

Editions of the famous letters are common, from that of Frankfort, 1683, to the three volumes of Réveillé-Parise, 1846—fourteen in all, and all imperfect, many garbled. A unique and priceless contribution, general and medical, to the history of the seventeenth century, "forming," as Triaire says, "a veritable diary improvised day by day, a mordant chronicle of the times by one of the most brilliant, the most alert, the most spirituel and the most satyric of the period." The worst possible luck has dogged all attempts to issue a definitive edition. Formey, of the Berlin Academy, in 1770, conceived the design to issue the correspondence complete with notes, but nothing came of it.

The edition of Réveillé-Parise, the only one of the nineteenth century, while a great improvement upon and much fuller than any other, had many errors, and perhaps deserved the severe handling given to it by Sainte-Beuve. MM. de Montaiglon and Tamisey de la Roque had collected material, collated the letters, and had one volume ready when, in 1895, a fire destroyed every page of their manuscripts. Not a whit discouraged by the ill-success of his predecessors, Dr. Paul Triaire, of Tours, already well-known for his biographical writings, undertook the task, and in 1907 issued one splendid volume containing the letters from 1830 to 1848. As illness overtook him, the work could not be completed, and the death of the accomplished editor has just been announced. It is a sad loss, a calamity in the world of letters.

21

Now for my protest: It is not often that a Frenchman makes a mistake in matters literary, but there is one, Pierre Pic, whom I would like to shake for the disappointment caused by a wretched abortion which has seen the light under the title of *Gui Patin, avec 74 portraits ou documents,* Paris, G. Steinheil, 1911. Pic has the shamefacedness to acknowledge that he does not know much of his subject—"Mais mon bagage à son sujet n'était pas lourd." This is evident. From two old editions which he has picked up he has sorted various extracts from the letters, but he has never even looked into—so he says, and one can well believe him—the edition of Réveillé-Parise, or the delightful first volume of Triaire with the early letters; and he appears to be ignorant of the important collection of letters in the Bibliothèque Nationale. One is not surprised at his judgement—"Gui Patin has been abominably over-rated. He is a bore . . ." It is a pity for M. Pic's reputation that he had not left him alone. Had he devoted a little appreciative study to his author, he might have come to the conclusion of his great countryman, Flourens, who saw the *man* through all his faults: "Gui Patin has really written nothing but his 'letters': and these 'letters,' in spite of a boldness of view which is sometimes extreme, in spite of language which is often common, in spite of many errors of judgement, of many prejudices against certain men—these letters are a brilliant expression of a proud and lofty soul, and in them he will live, for there is in them what never dies —style. Gui Patin is the most 'spirituel' doctor who has ever written, unless one includes Rabelais, in whom, however, medicine was hardly more than 'la qualité externe.' "

But the chief object of this note is to make an appeal, to express a hope, that the Paris Faculty will at once arrange for the completion of M. Triaire's edition. Much of the work has been done, and it should not be difficult to find someone with the necessary qualifications. They owe it to the memory of one of the greatest of their deans. When completed, an English edition should be forthcoming. From one of the old editions a translation has already been made by Dr. Blodgett, of Boston, who, at my request, has withheld it from the press awaiting the completion of Triaire's work.

XI. *George Bodington*

A GENERATION—two indeed—in advance of his day, George Bodington has at last come to his own, and is everywhere recognized as the pioneer of the open-air treatment of pulmonary tuberculosis. Not that he was the first to send consumptives into the open: Celsus speaks of sea voyages and the advantages of the climate of Egypt, and the horseback cure of Sydenham meant fresh air and exercise. But Bodington recognized that "to live in and breathe freely open air, without being deterred by the wind or weather, is one important and essential remedy in arresting tuberculosis."

I have long been looking for his rare *Essay on the treatment and cure of pulmonary consumption on principles natural, rational and successful,* London, 1840. A few weeks ago at Winchester, I met in consultation Dr. Arthur E. Bodington, and immediately asked what relation he was to the well-known physician of the same name. He replied, "His grandson." Then I said, "Well, perhaps you are the man who can give me a copy of his essay," and to my delight he had one to spare; and he not only gave me the original but also the very interesting reprint, which he issued in 1906, with a portrait and a sketch of the author.

A country practitioner, at first at Erdington, Bodington subsequently removed to Sutton Coldfield, where he had a private asylum, and where he lived until his death in 1882, in his eighty-third year. The period at which he wrote was not a very comfortable one for the poor consumptive. The prevalent method of treatment was to shut the patient up in a close room, excluding as far as possible the access of air, and to drug him with tartarized antimony and digitalis, alternating with occasional doses of calomel, and now and then to take a little blood! For all this Bodington substituted "fresh morning air, a good dinner to make him fat, an opium pill to make him sleep, and good wine to bring down his pulse." He had really the idea of sanatorium treatment. "I have taken for

23

the purpose a house in every respect adapted and near to my own residence for the reception of patients of this class, who may be desirous, or who are recommended to remove from their homes for the benefit of a change of air." He held that cold was never too severe for the consumptive patient: "The cooler the air which passes into the lungs the greater will be the benefit the patient will receive. Sharp, frosty days in the winter season are the most favourable. The application of cold, pure air to the interior surface of the lungs is the most powerful sedative that can be applied." He advocated riding or walking, according to the strength of the patient. Several cases are reported in the essay showing the very favourable results obtained by this treatment. As is often the case, his practice was better than his theory, for he had a belief that the disease was associated with impairment of the contractility of the lungs from loss of nervous power, consequent upon the presence of the tuberculous matter.

The house at Sutton Coldfield still stands, the prototype of the innumerable open-air sanatoria of to-day. A few years ago Dr. Lawrason Brown, of Saranac, made a pious pilgrimage to the place, and I am indebted to him for photographs of the house.

Bodington was severely criticized by his contemporaries, and he did not live to see the open-air method adopted, but has the great merit of being the first, or at any rate among the very first, to advocate rational and scientific treatment of pulmonary consumption.

XII. *Histoire de la Charité*

THE second part of Volume IV, of Lallemand's great work, Picard & Fils, Paris, is just to hand, covering the period from the sixteenth to the nineteenth century. There is nothing in literature of the same extent, as the work not only deals with the evolution of the hospital, but with all the accessory means of caring for the afflicted in mind and body. In progress for the past ten years, Volume I has dealt with the ancient civilizations; Volume II with the first nine centuries of the Christian era; Volume III with Europe in the Middle Ages, and Volume IV, both first and second parts, with the modern period to the nineteenth century. Though no book in English has quite the same scope, the *History of nursing,* by Miss Nutting and Miss Dock, gives much information not available elsewhere, and brings to date the story of training schools for nurses.

In the present volume, M. Lallemand deals with the story of the insane, dements, imbeciles, and epileptics. The famous Bedlam, in London, according to Burdett, was the first asylum for the insane established in Europe. This is a sad story, until one comes to the days of Pinel and of William Tuke. At the Bicêtre, in 1791, Pinel for the first time struck the chains off lunatics, from some indeed who had been in irons for ten, twenty, and even thirty years! Two years later he did the same at the Salpêtrière. From his prominent position as a teacher and the ability of his writings, he did more than any other man to introduce a humane treatment of the insane.

The organization in the sixteenth, seventeenth, and eighteenth centuries of the care of the blind, the deaf and dumb, and of foundlings, is considered in separate chapters.

A large part of the work is taken up with the consideration of the measures adopted for the care of the poor in various countries in Europe. The final chapters treat of the accessory means for helping the needy, such as the official pawn-shops, "Monts de

25

piétés." Apparently these were first organized at Rome in 1515, and spread throughout Italy and the Low Countries before they were established in Paris in 1611.

The extent and importance of the work may be judged from these brief memoranda. In Volume V, the author will consider the history of charity in America, in the ancient civilizations of India and among the Mahometans, and the question of slavery among the blacks.

XIII. *The School of Physic, Dublin**

To HAVE been selected to propose the toast of the evening I take as an honour to the university with which I am associated, Oxford, *mater studiorum* of these Isles in philosopy, theology, and medicine. In reality, the toast has already been proposed, and in fine form, by Dr. Kirkpatrick in the just issued *History of the School of Physic,* which the Provost and Fellows have so kindly distributed to their guests; and to enable you to drink the toast with sympathetic intelligence I should have to read to you the four hundred pages of his work. While Trinity College itself has had close affiliations with Cambridge, those of the School of Physic have been rather with Oxford. Stearne, the founder, was a close friend of Seth Ward, of Wadham College, and may have been a member of Boyle's "Invisible College" in those brilliant days when Wallis and Wilkins, Ward and Willis, Wren, Locke, Petty, and others "investigated nature by way of experiment." John Locke, the most famous name in English philosophy, and the great glory of the college with which I am connected, Christ Church, was a warm friend of the men who began this school—particularly of the Molyneauxs, William and Thomas: William, a philosopher of distinction, and the first man in this country, I believe, to see the capillary circulation; and Thomas, a distinguished physician, the first Irish medical baronet, and an early president of the College of Physicians.

An interesting manuscript in the Bodleian, in Locke's handwriting, contains a correspondence on the subject of vital statistics with two well-known Dublin physicians, Willoughby, a Fellow of Merton College, and Patrick Dun, the moving spirit of his day in the profession of this city—a wise, farseeing man, whose name is perpetuated in the hospital of this School.

*Toast proposed at the Graduates' Dinner, Bicentenary Celebration of the Trinity College Medical School, July 4th, 1912.

27

But Oxford's greatest gift to Ireland was her professor of anatomy and the vice-principal of Brasenose College, William Petty—philosopher, inventor, one of the founders of the Royal Society, promoter of this School of Physic, one of the founders of the science of political economy, author of the *Political Anatomy of Ireland*, and of the *Political Arithmetic;* but best remembered in Ireland in connexion with the famous Down Survey. Were there time, I should like to have dwelt upon some of the achievements of this extraordinary man, who came here as physician-general to the army, and who completed in thirteen months a survey which others had estimated would take as many years, and which is to-day "the legal record of the title on which half the land of Ireland is held."

Last year chance threw in my way the manuscript letter-book of Petty from 1666 to 1686, and the other evening I found, bound with them, an interesting manuscript of Petty dealing with the famous survey—the agreement with Fleetwood, the names of the officers, and the sums received from them, and the names of the men engaged in the work. The true bibliophile has a keen pleasure in seeing an important document in its proper home, and I have great pleasure, Mr. Provost, in asking you to place this in the library of Trinity College as a slight token of my appreciation of your warm reception of us on this memorable occasion.

We may pass over the dark days of the eighteenth century, in which the school experienced the trials and tribulations so common in the history of all institutions—days brightened, indeed, by the devotion and brilliant work of such men as Barry, Bryan Robinson, and Cleghorn. Then came the glorious period of the first half of the nineteenth century, when the Dublin School reached a zenith of world-wide fame in medicine, midwifery, and surgery. Medicine proper has passed through three phases of activity—the recognition of disease and the means for its cure, the discovery of its causes, and the measures for its prevention. It is the great merit of the Irish school to have taken a first place in the clinical study of disease.

You have had many men of the first rank as physicians—Barry, Cheyne, Adams, Whitley Stokes, Corrigan, Hudson, Lyons, Banks—to mention only those whose names I know best, but it is no disparagement to the memory of those distinguished men to say that the imperishable glory of your school is associated with

28

the names of Robert James Graves and William Stokes. Both were men of exceptional culture and refinement, devoted students of the Art, bedside teachers, whose influence is still potent, and authors who raised the fame of Irish medicine to a supreme height. I need say no more. Their works follow them, and are to-day full of lessons for those of us who realize that the best life of the teacher is in supervising the personal daily contact of patient with student in the wards.

This is a graduates' dinner, and at last I come to a part of the toast, which I know at first hand. Graduates of this school have been much in my life. To usher me into this breathing world one of them came many weary miles through the backwoods of Canada. Across his *tie,* as he called it, John King, M.A., T.C.D., birched into me small Latin and less Greek. I owe my start in the profession to James Bovell, a kinsman and devoted pupil of Graves, while my teacher in Montreal, Palmer Howard, lived, moved, and had his being in his old masters, Graves and Stokes.

From the days of Columba, the Irish of all classes have had a passion to perigrinate, and at every step in my career I have met your fellow graduates in Toronto, in Montreal, in many country districts of Canada, in the great cities of the United States, in lonely villages of Virginia and the Carolinas, and now in the very different surroundings of Harley Street and the pleasant villages of the Thames Valley—and everywhere the same intelligent and highly trained men, ever working with the Hippocratic spirit, *caute, caste et probe,* and ever leaving their patients if not in better health, at least in better spirits.

XIV. *Kelly's American Medical Biography*

WHAT more delightful in literature than biography? And yet, how uncertain and treacherous is the account which any man can give of another's life! And who is to be trusted to give a correct account of his own? Montaigne is the only great autobiographer; the only man whose spirit and pen make us feel that we know as much of him as any one of us could tell of himself; the only man we believe when he says, "I have either told all, or designed to tell all . . . I leave nothing to be desired or guessed at concerning me." However imperfectly told, the story of any life has an interest which appeals to us in direct proportion as we feel that brotherly sympathy with human effort, careless of the result, whether success or failure.

When my colleague, Howard Kelly, spoke of a scheme for a great work on American medical biography, I envied his extraordinary capacity for initiative and for work. Few men of his generation have known the profession of his own country so well, and with his gift for organization, and for getting good work out of others, I felt sure the plan would be successful. I remember that I urged him to take as a model the *Dictionary of National Biography,* and to choose subjects of the first rank only, and to have their lives written by various authors. The result is two big volumes in which American and Canadian medical biography is brought up-to-date. The work is well done and will be of permanent value for reference. But much more than this—it is of immense importance to have a sympathetic record of the men who have borne the burden and the heat in making the profession of the New World what it is to-day. There are lives we could have spared, of men who had attained great local prominence, but who contributed little to the common stock; but, in apologizing, Dr. Kelly remarks that some of these have influenced their fellows by a strong personality. The

30

best men are here and, with a few exceptions, the story of their lives is accurately told. With the *Index Catalogue* of the Surgeon-General's Library so accessible, the bibliographies could in many cases have been omitted. It is nice to have biographies of the men who laid so well the foundation stones of Canadian medicine— Holmes, Widmer, Campbell, Howard, Almon, Rolph, and others.

The volumes are full of surprises. Conrad Gesner is one of my heroes—physician, naturalist, lexicographer—one of the most fascinating figures in the profession of the sixteenth century, and it is intensely interesting to find that Dr. Abraham Gesner, a pioneer geologist of Nova Scotia and the discoverer of kerosene, was one of his descendants.

Very often I have come across the name of Mettauer, a most voluminous contributor to the older American periodicals. The story of his career is very extraordinary, as he appears to have been an ante-bellum predecessor of the Mayo brothers, having a surgical clinic of remarkable extent for those days, and for a country district in Virginia.

There are excellent sketches of the physician-naturalists and botanists, a group so dear to Dr. Kelly's heart, and the biographies of Agassiz, Asa Gray, and Morton, were of special interest to me.

There are a good many grievous omissions—the Jacksons, James, James, Jr., and J.B.S.; Henry I. Bowditch, and Henry J. Biglow, Boston men of the very first rank; Dickson, of Charlestown, S.C., one of the strongest writers of the profession; La-Roche, William Pepper, Senior, John Forsyth Meigs, the Rogers brothers of Philadelphia, and David Ramsay, the historian of the Revolution and of Washington—these should come in a second edition.

XV. *The Works of John Caius, M.D.*

IN CONNEXION with the four hundredth anniversary of the birth of John Caius, the governing body of his Cambridge college and the president and the fellows of the Royal College of Physicians have published an edition of his works (Cambridge University Press, price 18s net). Few men of his generation deserve to be held in more grateful remembrance, not so much for his works, though numerous and important, as for the character of the man and for what he did for the Royal College of Physicians and for his old college at Cambridge. Caius recognized the value of the organic life of the institutions of which he was a member. Of the London college he was president for many years, and he was "the inventor of that insignia of honour by which the president of the college is distinguished from the rest of the Fellows," and his silver caduceus is still carried by that officer. The annals of the college from 1555 to 1572 in manuscript appear in print in this volume for the first time. "He was so religious in observing the statutes of the college that, though old, he durst not absent himself from the college's *cunilia* without a dispensation." He restored the tomb of Linacre, the founder of the college, in St. Paul's Cathedral.

But Caius is most worthily remembered to-day by having, in Fuller's words, "improved the ancient Hall of Gonvil into a new college, of his own name," and to-day, as in the seventeenth century, he carries away, as Fuller has it, "the name of the college in common discourse." The charter of the new foundation, 1557, was accompanied with substantial gifts in lands and money, and two years later he became the master, though continuing his practice in London. While imbued with the new learning, Caius had a medieval mind, filled with the sense of the universal symbolism in material things. On the occasion of the feast, when refounding the college, he gave a cushion of reverence, a rod of prudence—a silver caduceus still in its possession—and a book of knowledge. And this is seen in the gates of the new court, which he built: one

32

low and little, *Humilitatis;* the next, a portico of handsome proportions, *Virtutis;* a third leading to the public schools, through which all had to pass for their degrees, was inscribed *Honoris.*

As an author, Caius occupies a distinguished place in the literature of the sixteenth century. A profound scholar, he has the rare distinction, unique perhaps for an Englishman, of having been elected "dialectes Graeci professor" at Padua, where he was the friend and colleague of Vesalius, with whom he lived for eight months. Following the example of Jerome Cardan, he wrote a work, *De libris propriis,* and gives seventy-two titles, "including sixteen original works, seven versions from the Greek and Latin, and ten commentaries, besides texts discovered, edited, and amended." A majority remained in manuscript, and have been lost. The medical work by which he is best known is "A boke or counseill against the disease commonly called the sweate or sweatyng sicknesse," an exceedingly rare work, one of the few of his original editions that I have never been able to procure. It is the first monograph in English on a separate disease. Caius had studied the fifth outbreak, a remarkable epidemic which began at Shrewsbury in 1551 and spread rapidly through England with a very high mortality. One cannot but wish that he had given us more symptoms and less treatment, but there are many shrewd observations. He urges the people to "seke out a good physicien and knowen to have skille, and at the leaste be so good to your bodies as you are to your hosen and shoes," for which the best makers are sought.

The little book on *British Dogs,* prepared for his friend, Conrad Gesner, has been often reprinted. His longest work is *De Antiquitate Cantabrigiensis,* "a fardell of strange antiquities," as one of his friends calls it. One Key or Caius of All Souls' College, Oxford, having extolled the antiquity of his University as founded by Greek philosophers, companions of Brutus, and restored by King Alfred, at the instigation of Archbishop Parker. John Caius asserted the antiquity of Cambridge and "with all the forms of antiquarian certainty and precision he established its foundation by one Cantaber 394 B.C. and in the year of the world 4300—gaining a priority of 1,267 years from Alfred."

He edited several of the books of Galen, for which he collated manuscripts in Italy, some of which are now in the library of Caius College.

33

It is sad to think that a man of his learning and devotion should have lost touch with the members of his own college, and that his last years should have been darkened with unseemly quarrels. Apparently he stuck to the old faith and was charged, not only with a "shew of a perverse stomach to the professions of the Gospel, but atheism." The fellows and students of his own college, aided by the Vice-Chancellor of the University, the Master of Trinity, and the Provost of King's, sacked his chambers and made a bonfire in the college court of the ornaments and ecclesiastical furniture and vestments. Fuller's characteristic comment upon him is: "We leave the heat of his faith to God's sole judgement, and the light of his good works to men's imitation."

XVI. *William Beaumont*

GENERATIONS of medical students have listened with keen interest to the tale of William Beaumont and his Canadian *voyageur*, Alexis St. Martin, one of the most instructive chapters in the history of physiology; but the story in full has lain buried in two old chests, the possession of Mrs. Keim, Dr. Beaumont's daughter. Some ten years ago she very kindly gave me access to some of these documents, which I used for an address on "A Pioneer American Physiologist," and now Dr. Jesse Myer, of St. Louis, has utilized them freely in the *Life and Letters of William Beaumont* (St. Louis, C. V. Mosby Co., 1912). The work is a model biography, in the preparation of which the author has gone to the original sources; and we have a picture drawn by a strong hand, with admirable taste and judgement.

It is a tribute to the care with which the old New England registers have been kept that the author has been able to trace the genealogy of William Beaumont to an ancestor of the same name who settled in Saybrook, Conn., about 1640. Born of a fine sturdy stock, with the "Wanderlust" still active, in 1806 the future physiologist, then just of age, refused the offer of a farm from his father and started north "with a horse and cutter, a barrel of cider and $100," seeking his fortune. At Champlain, in New York State, close to the Canadian border, he taught school for three years; at the end of which time he began the study of medicine under Dr. Chandler, of St. Albans, Vermont, with whom he served an apprenticeship for two years. From the note-books of this period Dr. Myer quotes a number of cases which show that the young student was already a keen observer.

In June, 1812, he presented himself for examination before the Medical Society of the State of Vermont, and received a license "as a judicious and safe practicioner in the different avocations of the medical profession." War with Great Britain had just been declared, and Beaumont was gladly received into the army at

35

Plattsburg, on December 22nd, as Surgeon's Mate. His diary of the expedition against Toronto—then Little York—and the capture of the fort, is full of interest, and here he had his first and very active experience in military surgery. He was on duty for nearly two years, and took part in the battle of Plattsburg in August, 1814.

Though still retaining his rank, he began practice with another army surgeon in Plattsburg, announcing that they had "commenced business in the line of their profession," in connexion with which they had also opened a general store. His note-books of this period show how carefully he kept the records of important cases.

Though very successful in practice, the longing for the old military life induced him, in 1830, to accept a commission as Post Surgeon, and he was detailed for service at Fort Mackinac (then on the far away north-west frontier), which he reached by way of the Great Lakes, taking a passage at Black Rock by the *Walk on the Water,* the first steamer on the upper lakes. His journals at this time are very full and valuable, giving an excellent description of the country.

At Mackinac, the centre of the trading posts in the North-West, in June, 1822, occurred the accident to the young French-Canadian, Alexis St. Martin, which gave Beaumont the opportunity of his life. The circumstances of the case are very fully given by Myer, and there is reproduced a most interesting facsimile of the first page of Beaumont's hospital record. It was not until 1825 that Beaumont realized the great importance of St. Martin for experimental purposes. Through the wound, by this time completely healed, he could look directly into the cavity of the stomach, and St. Martin had been taught to submit passively to almost any procedure.

The story of the famous experiments is in every work on physiology, but the details given by Dr. Myer enable us better to appreciate the troubles, worries, and difficulties with which Beaumont had to contend. The famous book on *Experiments and Observations on the Gastric Juice* appeared at Plattsburg in 1833. Badly printed, on poor paper, it is one of the most treasured of American medical monographs, copies of which are becoming increasingly scarce.

In 1834 Beaumont was transferred to Jefferson Barracks, St. Louis, which was to be his residence for the remainder of his life.

36

The following year he took part in the establishment of a School of Medicine in St. Louis, and was offered the Chair of Surgery. In 1840 he resigned his commission and began private practice. After a busy and prosperous life, Beaumont died in March, 1853, universally beloved in the community.

Alexis St. Martin returned to Canada, and spent the latter part of his life at St. Thomas de Joliette. In 1880 I saw a newspaper announcement of his death, and through Judge Baby and Dr. Duncan McCallum I tried hard to be allowed to secure the stomach for the Surgeon General's Museum at Washington, but the family resisted all requests. Judge Baby got for me the interesting photograph of St. Martin, in his eighty-first year, reproduced at page 299, showing the fistulous orifice.

Beaumont's observations settled many obscure points in the physiology of digestion, and one misses in Dr. Myer's book a critical discussion of the significance of his work, and its relation to more recent views. His experiments may be said to have settled finally the chemical nature of the digestive process, and among other important observations may be mentioned the confirmation of the discovery by Prout of the presence of hydrochloric acid in the gastric juice; the recognition that the essential elements of the gastric juice and the mucous secretion were separate; the establishment by direct observation of the profound influence of mental disturbances on the secretion of the gastric juice and on digestion; the fuller and more accurate comparative study of digestion in the stomach with digestion outside the body; the rapid disappearance of water from the stomach through the pylorus; the first comprehensive and full study of the motions of the stomach; the study of the digestibility of different articles of diet, which remains to-day one of the most important contributions ever made to practical dietetics; and the relation between the amount of food taken and the quantity of gastric juice secreted.

XVII. *The Young Laennec*

THE story of Laennec, discoverer of auscultation, and founder of modern clinical medicine, has been told and retold, but not all told. We know of the struggle, the great achievement, and the early death, but much remained jealously guarded by the family—"a very precious mine containing all kinds of treasures, but principally letters—numberless letters, from Laennec, from his father, from his grandfather, from his uncle—then college exercises; verses and humorous works; political and religious pamphlets; inedited notes on different subjects, medical and miscellaneous; prize-lists, diplomas, all sorts of official papers, genealogical documents, and even souvenirs." Some of these, so far as they relate to his life to 1806, are now laid before us in a charming brochure by Professor Alfred Rouxeau, of Nantes (*Laennec avant 1806,* Paris, Baillière & Fils).

Born in 1781, at Quimper, of strong Breton stock on both sides, neither the father nor the mother of Théophile appear to have shown any special ability; the former, indeed, had careless talents, but no persistency, while the mother died before the boy had reached his sixth year. The outlook would have been dark for her motherless children, had not the Uncle William, a professor in the medical faculty at Nantes, and at the time rector of the university, offered them a home, and an ideal one it proved to be for the young Théophile.

Guillaume-François Laennec, a cultured, highly trained physician "with a volcanic head, but a warm heart," quickly saw that his nephew was a boy of more than ordinary parts, and gave him the best training Nantes could afford. Keen at his books, but keen also at all games, the young student made rapid progress, and his studies were continued even during the horrors of the civil war. The ghastly guillotine was erected under the very windows of their house, to the basement and back rooms of which they had to flee to escape the shrieks of the victims and the noise of their falling heads! The uncle himself was a suspect, but doctors' heads had a value even in those terrible days. It is an extraordinary fact that the college (school) did not close, and the studies of "le jeune citoyen Laennec," and of his brothers were not interrupted, but they had to participate in the famous Fête of the Supreme Being. Laennec became interested in Natural History, and made long excursions into the country to collect insects, plants, and birds.

In 1795, at the early age of fourteen years and seven months, he began the study of medicine and was officially attached to one of the military hospitals as "surgeon of the third class," a position corresponding to that of surgical dresser. The civil war had necessitated the creation of new military hospitals, and the work of the medical school at the Hôtel Dieu (now the Temple of Humanity) had been interrupted, but dissections were continued at the Hôtel Dieu in a room beneath and communicating with one of the wards. Physics and chemistry were taught at the "École centrale."

The devoted uncle watched with pride the growing talents of the young student, though at times distressed by his irrepressible tendency to compose verses and to spend long hours in his natural history studies. In the letters to his father and stepmother a delightful picture is given of the inner life of the lad at this period, with its hopes and disappointments. Money was scarce, the times were perilous; it was difficult to get the necessaries of life, and such luxuries as dancing and flute playing did not appeal to the hard-pressed uncle. The young Laennec found it hard to get anything from his ne'er-do-well father, to whom, after an absence of nine years, he paid a visit at Quimper (1797). The stepmother wished him to take up some business, and it was only a strong appeal on the part of Dr. Laennec that frustrated her designs: "For God's sake let him come back to me as I sent him to you, good, gentle and studious; let him pursue in peace a course of study which is good for his health, sufficient for his fortune and honourable for his reputation"—and he had his way. The lad walked to and from Quimper to Nantes in four and a half days at the rate of about forty-one kilometres a day. There are sad letters telling of many trials and worries, lack of proper clothing, no money for books, or for his fees, and the uncle too hard-up to do anything, and the father too careless to answer letters. After following for five years the courses at the Hôtel Dieu and the work at the military hospital, Laennec passed the examination for the grade of "Officier de santé."

In 1800 a widespread insurrection occurred in the west, and for a time he served with the regular army in the field. Then followed a period of great anxiety and depression. The desire of his life had been to finish at Paris, but there were no funds, and a sixth year of hope deferred had to be spent at Nantes. At last the fledgling took flight and, in 1801, with a light heart and light pocket, with only eight hundred francs, the young Théophile set out to conquer Paris. In those terrible days Nantes had been a hard school, but he had laid a good foundation in practical work, he had picked up a fair education, and above all he had developed an intense love for his work. He had given play to a poetic temperament and Professor Rouxeau gives a number of small poems, some of which indicate that a certain "Nisa" had stirred his Breton heart. With a group of old Nantes students and friends he was soon at home in Paris, and at once attached himself to the Charité Hospital, where Corvisart had already revolutionized the teaching of medicine. To-day Paris still follows this great master's method—the morning ward visit, and afterwards the amphitheatre lecture. We get a good idea of the state of medicine in Paris at this time from Joseph Frank's *Reise nach Paris und London* (Wien, 1805). Lectures on the doctrines of Hippocrates were still given three times a week, and one morning at the Hôtel Dieu he saw thirty patients bled out of the one hundred and forty-two in the wards of Bosquillon; but Corvisart was effecting a revolution, and teaching men to observe and compare at bedside and in dead-house. Here, too, was working the man who was to influence Laennec strongly, Bayle; and for a short time he had the inestimable advantage of the instruction and example of Bichat. At the École Pratique he became associated with Dupuytren, and others of his teachers were Pinet and Cabanis. A good short-hand writer, he utilized this gift to make careful notes of lectures and reports on his cases.

In the *Journal de Médecine* in 1802 appeared his first important communication—"Histoires d'Inflammation de Peritoine," a clinical and pathological study on an affection at that time but little known.

In 1802, largely through the influence of Bayle, he became converted, and in 1803 joined the famous religious fraternity, the Congregation. In the letters to his father and uncle we can follow the progress of his scientific work, and papers appeared on the arachnoid, on a synovial membrane, etc.

In 1803, at the concours for the prizes at the School of Medicine, Laennec had a double triumph, taking those for medicine and surgery, and both in money—a welcome addition to his ever slender purse. One can imagine the delight of the uncle at Nantes —"He is a treasure, that boy"—who predicted a professorship in a few years.

Leaving Nantes with a good knowledge of Latin, English, and German, Laennec worked hard at Greek, and in 1804 wrote his doctor's thesis on the doctrine of Hippocrates. A partially written "Traité sur l'Anatomie Pathologique" of that period remained in manuscript until edited by Cornil in 1884. Working at clinical medicine and pathological anatomy, writing for the journals, an active participant in the medical societies, the young Breton of twenty-five had made a strong impression on his contemporaries; but life was still a struggle. He had begun to practice, and—have courage young men!—had only taken one hundred and fifty francs in his first year and four hundred in the second. But he had much capital in his brain-pan, and how the promise of his youth was fulfilled Professor Rouxeau has reserved for another volume.

XVIII. *Mediaeval Medicine*

A BOOK has recently appeared, which gives a good picture of the state of medicine in the fourteenth century—*John of Gaddesden and the Rosa Medicinae* (Oxford Press). Dr. Cholmeley has here sketched the life and work of the earliest teacher of medicine in England. Gaddesden entered Merton College about 1294 and, after finishing the course of Arts, studied medicine for a period of six years. "The candidate had to have 'read' one book of the Tegni, i.e. τέγνη of Galen, or one book of the Aphorisms of Hippocrates, *pro majori parte*. These were to serve as far as 'theory went.' As regarded practical medicine, the candidate must have read one book of the *Regimentum Acutorum* of Hippocrates, or the *Liber Febrium* of Isaac, or the *Antidotarum* of Nicolaus (Praepositus, of Salerno). A candidate must also have responded to the Masters Regent in the faculty for two years." So far as we know neither dissection nor hospital work was demanded.

John of Gaddesden taught in the university, and in the seventh year of his "lecture" wrote the treatise known as *Rosa Medicinae* or, as it is more often called, *Rosa Anglicae*. After a far-fetched comparison of the five parts of his book with the five appendages of the rose, he modestly goes on to say: "And as the rose overtops all flowers, so this book overtops all treatises on the practice of medicine, and it is written for both poor and rich surgeons and physicians, so that there shall be no need for them to be always running to consult other books, for here they will find plenty about all curable disease both from the special and the general point of view."

Largely a compilation from Greek, Arabian, and Jewish physicians, the chief value of this work is in the personal observations which show the author to have been a shrewd, capable man, though not a little given to boasting and to doubtful practices. Some of the pen pictures of disease are admirable, e.g., dropsy, and the description of paracentesis for ascites might be copied

42

into a modern manual—the hole in the skin and in the peritoneum are to be at different levels, the fluid is to be drawn off slowly, never all at once "lest the patient die suddenly." It is curious to note the recommendation of a diet with very little salt. The *Rosa Anglicae* is most often quoted now in connexion with the red-light treatment of small-pox, with which Gaddesden cured the king's son. It was not original, but was an old woman's remedy of the time. An appalling number of medicines were used, and he gives a selection of charms and prayers. Curiously enough he is silent on astrological matters. Avicenna and Galen are the most frequently quoted authors.

Dr. Cholmeley has added chapters on the mediaeval physician and on the study of medicine at Oxford in the fourteenth century, and has given a translation of the *Isagoge* of Joannitus, an Arabian physician of the ninth century, which formed an introduction to Galen's *Ars parva,* one of the most popular of the textbooks in the Middle Ages.

It is very difficult for us to appreciate, still more so to understand, the mediaeval mind. To those interested, let me recommend Henry Osborn Taylor's *Mediaeval Mind* (Macmillan and Co.). The author, "a scholar, and a ripe and good one," has a warm sympathy and a keen art, which enable him to paint for us a vivid and intelligent picture of the period.

XIX. *Robert Fletcher*

ANY time during the past twenty-five years special visitors to the great medical library in Washington have been received in a room next to that of the principal librarian, and have had their wants and wishes attended to by a courtly and learned man who has just passed away in his ninetieth year. Surrounded by books of reference, volumes of the Index Catalogue, tables strewn with proof sheets and the newest journals, Dr. Robert Fletcher looked like a student of the old days. But he was more: he had two essential qualities of a great librarian—kindliness of manner, and a genuine interest in books. With Dr. John Billings, and the successive Surgeons-General, he has had an important share in two of the greatest bibliographical works of modern times, the *Index Catalogue* and the *Index Medicus*. But first a word or two of biography.

Born in Bristol, March 6th, 1823, the son of an accountant, after a few years at the Bristol Medical School, Dr. Fletcher went to the London Hospital, and in 1844 became a member of the Royal College of Surgeons. In 1847 he went to the United States and settled in Cincinnati, where he practised medicine for some years. On the outbreak of the Civil War he joined the 1st Regiment of Ohio Volunteers, served through the war and was breveted lieutenant-colonel, and afterwards colonel, for faithful and meritorious service. In 1871 he was ordered to Washington and was at first attached to the Provost-marshal's office, and took part in the preparation in 1875 of the volumes of *Anthropometric Statistics.*

In 1876 he was transferred to the Surgeon-general's library. Here he became associated with Dr. John Billings, who had already begun the preparation of the famous *Index Catalogue.* Nothing comparable with this colossal work had ever been undertaken before in the history of the profession. Not only is it a printed catalogue of the books in the library, but it is an index of all the journal articles. Since 1880 thirty-two volumes have been published, each containing nearly a thousand pages and the total

44

sum of 286,255 book titles, and 1,006,355 journal articles. Not so much the vaulting ambition that promoted the Index excites our wonder, as that men could be found with the energy and perseverance year by year to carry it out. But in Dr. John Billings, no ordinary mortal, are combined tenacity of purpose, good judgement, and painstaking accuracy. He was fortunate to secure as his lieutenant Dr. Fletcher, and, in the preface to the first volume, acknowledged specially his valuable assistance, without which the work could not have been carried on. After Dr. Billings' resignation the brunt of the work fell on Dr. Fletcher.

As a book of reference the *Index Catalogue* is of incalculable value, and not enough used by the profession. Any one in doubt about an obscure case, or if a biographical or bibliographical reference is needed, has only to turn up a volume in one or other of the series, and the chances are a hundred to one that he will find helpful information. And a remarkable feature is its accuracy. It is the rarest occurrence to find typographical or other errors.

In 1879 Dr. Billings began the publication of the *Index Medicus* with Dr. Fletcher as his co-editor, and for the last nine years Dr. Fletcher has been editor-in-chief.

After the organization of the Johns Hopkins Medical School, we asked Dr. Fletcher to give lectures on Medical Jurisprudence, a subject in which he was greatly interested. He also took part in the organization of the Historical Club at the hospital, and in this way, year by year, we learned to know him well, and to appreciate his delightful personality.

One of two things happens after sixty, when old age takes a fellow by the hand. Either the rascal takes charge as general factotum, and you are in his grip body and soul; or you take him by the neck at the first encounter, and after a good shaking make him go your way. This Dr. Fletcher did so successfully that with all that should accompany old age, he carried on his work faithfully to the very end, reading proofs to within a few days of his death. Of few men could it be said more truthfully, "He saw life steadily and saw it whole." As his friend and collaborator, Dr. Garrison wrote me: "Even on his grey days his wonderful will-power and stoicism are something to command admiration. You have probably heard his favourite *argumentum ad baculinum* for any bodily complaint—'treat it with contempt.' " And this is the best lesson of his long and useful life.

xx. *Jaques Bénigne Winslow*

His foramen and his ligament have made at least the name of this great Danish (and French) anatomist familiar to every student of medicine. The chief facts of his busy life are in all the biographies; but he left on record his own story, which has been carefully preserved in the Mazarin Library, Paris, and recently edited by his countryman Vilhelm Maar, to whom I am indebted for a copy. (*L'Autobiographie de Jaques Bénigne Winslow,* publiée par Vilhelm Maar. Octave Doin and Fils, Paris; Vilhelm Tryde, Copenhague MCMXII.)

Born in 1669, the son of a Protestant pastor, and great-nephew of the famous Sténon, Winslow began his studies under the direction of his father, and then proceeded to the École de Saint Canut, from which he passed to the University of Copenhagen, intending to study theology. A new student was made *Civis Academicus* with singular and sometimes brutal formalities by his fellows, and the description he gives reminds one of the ceremonies in vogue when I was a medical student at McGill in connexion with the so-called "footing supper." He soon came under the influence of Caspar Bartolin and Jacobaeus, professors in the medical faculty, and deserted theology for the study of anatomy. After graduating he attracted the attention of M. Moth (at the time secretary of state) who had at one time studied medicine, and had been a friend of Sténon, and who arranged a royal travelling fellowship for him.

In 1697, in company with a friend, he proceeded to Holland, where he studied for some time with Bidloo, Ruysch, and Rau. He speaks of the wonderful skill of Ruysch in the preparation of specimens, and was shown two entire bodies of infants perfectly preserved by some secret method. He seems to have seen everything that was of importance in Holland, and was much impressed by the practical advantages offered for the study of anatomy and surgery—*audio, video, palpo,* he says.

46

In June, 1698, he arrived in Paris, with which city his life was henceforward to be so intimately associated. Here, under the influence of Duverney, the well-known anatomist, he devoted his time to dissections and to surgery. But he had always retained an interest in theology, and this was increased by the arrival in Paris of a compatriot, M. Worm, a student of the subject. Several books of the illustrious Bossuet had fallen into Winslow's hands, and he and his young fellow-countryman decided to have a discussion, or conference, on the doctrines of the Roman Church. Winslow took the Roman side, and in the preparation for the discussion became intensely interested in Bossuet. The upshot was that he decided to consult the famous theologian on the subject of his doubts. The most interesting, and a very large, part of the autobiography is taken up with the story of his conversion. After many interviews with Bossuet he was received into the Church of Rome. As a special Danish scholar and a Protestant of note, his conversion attracted a good deal of attention, and the ceremony of his abjuration in the chapel of Germigny was performed in the presence of a number of distinguished people. Bossuet administered the rite of baptism, and added to his name Jaques that of Bénigne. Naturally the news of his conversion upset his family and friends in Denmark, and was a sore grief to his old father, to whom he was deeply attached.

Then began a long struggle for success in Paris. Duverney befriended him, and Bossuet appears to have helped him in every possible way. He was elected physician to the Hôtel Dieu, and in 1710 to the Bicêtre, and in 1721 he was made one of the professors of surgery. Meanwhile, he had devoted himself to the study of anatomy, and in 1732 appeared his well-known *Exposition Anatomique,* one of the most popular text-books of the eighteenth century, which was translated into many languages, and raised his reputation to that of one of the first anatomists of Europe. He had the misfortune not to succeed his old teacher Duverney in the chair of anatomy and surgery at the Jardin du Roi. In 1745 he inaugurated the new amphitheatre of anatomy of the faculty, still in existence and known as the amphitheatre of Winslow.

In addition to his well-known *Anatomy,* he wrote many monographs, most of which are published in the transactions of the Académie des Sciences. He had not much success as a surgeon or practitioner. With a timid nature he lacked confidence in himself;

47

and mentions in his autobiography that he had an almost insurmountable difficulty in performing even the minor operation of venesection. It is reported that he was so fearful that he would not order two ounces of manna without a prayer. He never returned to his native land, and even refused to visit the King of Denmark when dangerously ill in 1730.

The autobiography only extends to 1704. It is a pity that so much of it is occupied with theological discussions, some of which were carried on with his father. Winslow was much behind his age in certain matters, and had the old-fashioned idea that certain mental affections were possessions of the devil. He died in 1760, and was buried in the church of Saint-Benoit. His monument at present rests in the court of the Convent of Saint-Étienne du Mont.

Winslow cut a great figure in his day and generation, and had a wide reputation as a teacher and anatomist. It is interesting that his religious career should have somewhat resembled that of his more famous countryman and kinsman, Sténon. He appears to have been, in the words inscribed on this tomb, *vir aeque verax et pius.*

XXI. *Aristotle–Greek Thinkers*
by Gomperz, Vol. IV.

READERS of my occasional addresses will have noted frequent references to the work of Professor Gomperz on *Greek Thinkers,* Volume IV of which has just appeared. To young men with leisure, young practitioners in the waiting stage, who wish to keep the dough of their minds leavened, let me commend these volumes. An hour a day, or less, for a year, with a note book, and I can promise the best of company and a stimulating diet, full of intellectual hormones. If it be true that a man is born a Platonist or an Aristotelian, my congenital bias was towards the great idealist, but without, I fear, the proper mental equipment; the cares of this world and the deceitfulness of my studies have driven me into the camp of the Stagirite. And it is a glorious tribe, to be sealed of which, even as a humblest member, one should be proud. In the first circle of the *Inferno,* Virgil leads Dante into a wonderful company, the philosophic family who look with reverence on "the Master of those who know"—and so with justice has Aristotle been regarded for these twenty-three centuries*. No man has ever swayed such an intellectual empire—in logic, metaphysics, rhetoric, psychology, ethics, poetry, politics and natural history, in all a creator and in all still a master. The history of the human mind offers no parallel to the career of the great Stagirite.

It is as a biologist that Aristotle has a special interest for us. Professor D'Arcy Thompson, who dealt recently with this side of his activities, thus sums up his attitude as a student of life:

"But he was, and is, a very great naturalist. When he treats of natural history, his language is our language, and his methods and problems are well nigh identical with our own. He had familiar knowledge of a thousand varied forms of life, of bird and beast, of plant and creeping thing. He was careful to note their least details of outward structure, and curious to probe by dissection into their parts within. He studied the metamorphoses of gnat and butterfly, and opened the bird's egg to find the mystery of incipient life in

*"The good collector of the qualities," Dioscorides, Hippocrates, Avicenna, and Galen were the medical members of the group.

the embryo chick. He recognized great problems of biology that are still ours to-day, problems of heredity, of sex, of nutrition and growth, of adaptation, of the struggle for existence, of the orderly sequence of Nature's plan. Above all, he was a student of Life itself. If he was a learned anatomist, a great student of the dead, still more was he a lover of the living. Evermore his world is in movement. The seed is growing, the heart beating, the frame breathing. The ways and habits of living things must be known: how they work and play, love and hate, feed and procreate, rear and tend their young; whether they dwell solitary, or in more and more organized companies and societies. All such things appeal to his imagination and his diligence. Even his anatomy becomes at once *anatomia animata,* as Haller, poet and physiologist, described the science to which he gave the name of 'physiology.' "*

Before Aristotle there were other great students of nature among the Greeks, but he first taught men to look upon nature's naked loveliness—to use Shelley's phrase. The noble character of the man as a devoted husband and father, and as a master, are illustrated in his will, of which Gomperz gives an analysis. But the biologist did not escape altogether from the idealism of his great master, Plato. On the grave of his first wife he offered sacrifices as to a heroine, and a votive offering was to be presented in gratitude for the escape from danger of Nicanor, his son-in-law, who was to be "father and brother in one" to his younger children.

The son of a physician, Aristotle saw, as no one had seen before, the value of science in medicine. The following sentences, with which the *De Respiratione* concludes, might have been written to-day: "But health and disease also claim the attention of the scientist, and not merely of the physician, in so far as an account of their causes is concerned. The extent to which these two differ and investigate diverse provinces must not escape us, since facts show that their inquiries are, to a certain extent, at least conterminous. For physicians of culture and refinement make some mention of natural science, and claim to derive their principles from it, while the most accomplished investigators into nature generally push their studies so far as to conclude with an account of medical principles."**

*On Aristotle as a Biologist, by D'Arcy W. Thompson, Oxford, February 14th, 1913, p. 14.
**The Works of Aristotle, translated by J. A. Smith and W. D. Ross. Part I. Parva Naturalia. p.480 b., Oxford, 1908.

XXII. *Dr. Slop*

AT LAST some one has done justice to John Burton the man-mid-wife of York, so cruelly held up to ridicule by Stern in *Tristram Shandy* as Dr. Slop; and it has been well done by Alban Doran in the current number (January, February), of the *British Journal of Obstetrics and Gynoecology.*

It is surprising that Dr. Ferriar, the distinguished Manchester physician, who exposed so pitilessly the plagiarisms of *Tristram Shandy* in the *Illustrations of Sterne* (1798), did not devote a chapter to his contemporary, Dr. Burton. The only man I know who speaks a good word for him is his townsman, James Atkinson, the author of the *Medical Bibliography, A and B* (1834), the most fascinating book on the subject ever written. In a character-istically anecdotal sketch, he comes out bravely in Burton's de-fence. Certainly he was a man of parts, not only a distinguished physician, but the author of a celebrated work, still an authority, on the antiquities of Yorkshire.

Burton was born in 1710, studied first at St. John's College, Cambridge, and afterwards at Leyden, under Boerhaave. He be-gan practice in York, where he seems early to have acquired the nickname of "Dr. Slop." He practised as a physician and a mid-wife. As a strong Tory, Burton quarrelled with Archdeacon Sterne, uncle of Laurence, and in 1745, at the time of the Jacobe-an rising, was arrested. Sympathy with Prince Charlie cost him two years in prison, and a libellous portrait in *Tristram Shandy.* Shandy Senior had read much, and was full of fads, one of which was the terrible danger to the delicate structure of the brain in the process of delivery. When his son and heir was ready to appear, the father would very much rather have had a Caesarean Section made so as to spare the child's brain. For safety Dr. Slop was sent for. (Burton had already written his best known medical work—*Essay towards a complete new system of Midwifery,* 1751). How Dr. Slop forgot his obstetrical bag, and how Obadiah, who was sent for it, knotted it so that Slop cut his thumb in solving the knot

51

with a pen-knife, how he cursed Obadiah with the famous curse of Bishop Ernulphus, may be laughed over in Sterne's memorable story.

Mr. Alban Doran, discussing the type of forceps used by Burton, brings out a number of new points, the most interesting of which is that the forceps at present preserved in York, which was in Burton's possession, is not the forceps which he invented and which goes by his name. It is, however, the one which he actually used, and the one with which, we may suppose, he broke the bridge of Tristram's nose, to the unutterable grief of Shandy Senior.

Doran gives an account of the quarrel between Burton and Smellie, the well-known obstetrical author, whom Burton convicted of a curious mistake. He thought the Latin name of a calcified foetus was an author. In *Tristram Shandy* (Bk. 2, Chap. xix.), Sterne refers to this mistake in which Smellie regards *Lithopadus* as author of a book "De Partu Difficili," but in a foot-note a correction is made, as Sterne had seen the published letter of Burton to Smellie.

Burton's *Midwifery* was popular and was translated into French. He wrote also a treatise on the *Non-Naturals,* and minor essays. Of his work on the *Antiquities of Yorkshire,* only one volume appeared.

Through Burton's influence and energy, the York Infirmary was founded, and this is perhaps his best memorial.

Doran's estimate of him may be quoted: "Dr. John Burton was an able scientific obstetrician, and his 'Essay' shows that he was a man of practical experience. He was also a prominent citizen of York, the founder of its hospital, a noble philanthropic work, the benefits of which are continued to this day. Besides, this famous obstetrician was a highly distinguished antiquary, author of a standard work still much prized by librarians. Doctors and archaeologists quoted above have alike testified to his merits. In days when the man-midwife was looked down upon, Burton lived, a gentleman and a scholar." And I may add he was a worthy student of the great Boerhaave, whose *Life* (London, 1743) I believe is from his pen.

XXIII. *John Shaw Billings*

AMONG the men of our profession made distinguished by the American Civil War, Dr. Billings takes an unusual position. One hears sometimes that the career of the Army Surgeon offers small scope to a man of capability and energy, but to this the life of Dr. Billings is a strong contradiction. Without special advantages in early life, and without special opportunities during the war itself, he showed such capacity for work and for organization that when peace was declared he was one of the fortunate ones to be selected to utilize the enormous materials that had accumulated during the war. Plenty of opportunities now came to him, and a great one in connection with the Surgeon-General's Library. There have been great bibliographers in medicine since the famous Conrad Gesner wrote his *Bibliotheca Universalis* in 1545, but no one has ever undertaken and carried to completion so monumental a work of this character as the *Index Catalogue*.

Dr. Billings was born in 1839, and graduated from the Medical College of Ohio in 1860; after a session as demonstrator of anatomy he joined the Northern army and served throughout the Civil War, at the conclusion of which he was Medical Inspector of the army of the Potomac. He then became attached to the Surgeon-General's Office in Washington. In utilizing the enormous clinical and statistical material of the war, a serious difficulty arose owing to lack of the necessary works of reference. Surgeon-General Hammond had already started a library in connexion with his office and this formed the beginning of the now famous collection. Dr. Billings was put in charge of the few hundred volumes and given a free hand. With a large annual appropriation, Europe was ransacked for books and files of journals, and the library grew with extraordinary rapidity. In this bibliographical work, the late Dr. Windsor of Manchester acted as his friend and adviser. In the last report, October, 1912, the library is said to contain 178,741 bound volumes and 317,740 pamphlets. The collection is extraordinarily rich in old fifteenth century works, and particularly in

53

the journal literature of the world. Owing to the liberality and freedom with which successive Surgeons-General have allowed its treasures to be utilized, the library has had an important influence upon the medical profession in the United States.

In 1876, as the library began to grow, the question of a printed catalogue was discussed, and a *specimen fasciculus* was distributed for purposes of criticism. The work progressed slowly, but in 1880 Volume I of an *Index Catalogue* was printed, containing nearly a thousand pages. As subject and author catalogue it was immediately recognized that such a publication would be of the greatest help, but few at that time thought that a work on so vast a scale should be kept up. The literature of every subject was given with extraordinary fullness, though representing only the material available in the library; thus in Volume I under Aneurysm there were some 70 pages of references. Year by year the work progressed, and the first series of sixteen volumes was completed in 1895. Dr. Billings had a happy faculty for choosing able assistants, and he early had the good fortune to associate with him Dr. Robert Fletcher, whose death was noticed in the *Journal* a couple of months ago. The first volume of the second series was published in 1896, and Volume XVII of Series II has just been issued. The remarkable growth of medical literature is well illustrated by comparing the references on Syphilis in Volume XIV of the first series and Volume XVII of the second; in the one there were 109 pages, and in the other 207.

It was always a marvel to Dr. Billings' friends how year by year he kept up the publication of the *Index Catalogue,* but he used laughingly to say that it was only a matter of organization. He read every page of the proofs, and the singular accuracy which characterizes the work is due to Dr. Fletcher and himself. As an outgrowth of this library work the *Index Medicus* of current literature was started by Dr. Billings and continued, after his death, by Dr. Fletcher.

Early in his career Dr. Billings became interested in public health and in hospital organization, and was in charge of the preparation of the vital statistics for both the tenth and eleventh census of the United States. Of the Johns Hopkins Hospital Trust Dr. Billings was appointed adviser; he drew up the plans for the hospital and was active in getting it organized. An important interview I had with him illustrates the man and his methods. Early in

54

the spring of 1889 he came to my rooms in Walnut Street, Philadelphia. We had heard a great deal about the Johns Hopkins Hospital, and, knowing that he was virtually in charge, it flashed across my mind that he had come in connexion with it. Without sitting down, he asked me abruptly, "Will you take charge of the Medical Department of the Johns Hopkins Hospital?" Without a moment's hesitation I answered "Yes." "See Welch about the details; we are to open very soon. I am very busy today; good morning"; and he was off, having been in my room not more than a couple of minutes.

In the early days of the hospital, Dr. Billings' counsel was always sought, and the growth of the school was a matter of pride to him. For many years he was lecturer on the history of medicine. In 1891 he accepted the professorship of hygiene at the University of Pennsylvania, and became director of its new laboratory of hygiene. In 1896 he became director of the New York Public Library under the Astor, Lenox and Tilden foundations, and the crowning work of his life has been to consolidate these collections, and to see them housed in the magnificent building that was opened two years ago. The extent of the library may be gathered from the fact that it has more than 2,000,000 volumes and upwards of fifty branch libraries, with a staff of 1,002 persons.

In the foundation of the Carnegie Institution in Washington, Dr. Billings took an active share, and for years he was chairman of its board.

Dr. Billings was the author of many works on vital and social statistics, on bibliography and on hygiene. Honorary degrees were conferred on him by Edinburgh, Oxford, Dublin, Munich, Harvard, Yale, and other universities. His two strong qualities were a capacity for work and for organization. He worked easily without fuss or effort, but incessantly. He had an equable temperament, and took the accidents and worries of life in a philosophic spirit. Of late years he was often in the hands of the surgeons, on several occasions for very serious operations, which he bore with his characteristic equanimity.

xxiv. *Israel and Medicine**

IN ESTIMATING the position of Israel in the human values we must remember that the quest for righteousness is oriental, the quest for knowledge occidental. With the great prophets of the East—Moses, Isaiah, Mahomet—the word was "Thus saith the Lord"; with the great seers of the West, from Thales and Aristotle to Archimides and Lucretius, it was "What says Nature?" They illustrate two opposite views of man and his destiny—in the one he is an *"angelus sepultus"* in a muddy vesture of decay; in the other, he is the "young light-hearted master" of the world, in it to know it, and by knowing to conquer.

Modern civilization is the outcome of these two great movements of the mind of man, who to-day is ruled in heart and head by Israel and by Greece. From the one he has learned responsibility to a Supreme Being, and the love of his neighbour, in which are embraced both the Law and the Prophets; from the other he has gathered the promise of Eden to have dominion over the earth on which he lives. Not that Israel is all heart, nor Greece all head, for in estimating the human value of the two races, intellect and science are found in Jerusalem and beauty and truth at Athens, but in different proportions.

It is a striking fact that there is no great oriental name in science—not one to be put in the same class with Aristotle, with Hippocrates, or with a score of Grecians. We do not go to the Bible for science, though we may go to Moses for instruction in some of the best methods in hygiene. Nor is the Talmud a fountainhead in which men seek inspiration to-day as in the works of Aristotle. I do not forget the saying:

> "In uns'rem Talmud kann man Jedes lesen,
>
> Und Alles ist schon einmal dagewesen."

With much of intense interest for the physician, and in spite of some brave sayings about the value of science, there is not in it

*Remarks made at the dinner commemorating the Twenty-Fifth Anniversary of the Jewish Historical Society, London, April 27, 1914.

the spirit of Aristotle or of Galen. It is true we find there one of the earliest instances in literature of an accurate diagnosis confirmed post mortem. A sheep of the Rabbi Chabiba had paralysis of the hind legs. Rabbi Jemar diagnosed ischias, or arthritis, but Rabbina who was called in said that the disease was in the spinal marrow. To settle the dispute the sheep was killed, and Rabbina's diagnosis was confirmed.

In the early Middle Ages the Jewish physicians played a role of the first importance as preservers and transmitters of ancient knowledge. With the fall of Rome the broad stream of Greek science in western Europe entered the mud of mediaevalism. It filtered through in three streams—one in South Italy, the other in Byzantium, and a third through Islam. At the great school of Salernum in the tenth, eleventh and twelfth centuries, we find important Jewish teachers; Copho II wrote the *Anatomia Porci,* and Rebecca wrote on fevers and the foetus. Jews were valued councillors at the court of the great Emperor Frederick.

With the Byzantine stream the Jews seem to have had little to do, but the broad, clear stream which ran through Islam is dotted thickly with Hebrew names. In the eastern and western Caliphates and in North Africa were men who to-day are the glory of Israel, and bright stars in the medical firmament. Three of these stand out preëminent. The writings of Isaac Judaeus, known in the Middle Ages as Monarcha Medicorum, were prized for more than four centuries. He had a Hippocratic belief in the powers of nature and in the superiority of prevention to cure. He was an optimist and held strongly to the Talmudic precept that the physician who takes nothing is worth nothing.

Rabbi ben Ezra was a universal genius and wanderer, whose travels brought him as far as England. His philosophy of life Browning has depicted in the well-known poem, whose beauty of diction and clarity of thought atone for countless muddy folios. But the prince among Jewish physicians, whose fame as such has been overshadowed by his reputation as a Talmudist and philosopher, is the Doctor Perplexorum—*dux,* director, demonstrator, *neutrorum dubitantium et errantium*—Moses Maimonides.

Cordova boasts of three of the greatest names in the history of Arabian medicine: Avenzoar, Albucasis, and Averroes (Avenzoar is indeed claimed to be a Jew). Great as is the fame of Averroes as the commentator and transmitter of Aristotle to scholastic

57

Europe, his fame is enhanced as the teacher and inspirer of Moses ben Maimon. Exiled from Spain, this great teacher became in Egypt the Thomas Aquinas of Jewry, the conciliator of the Bible and the Talmud with the philosophy of Aristotle. He remains one of Israel's great prophets, and while devoted to theology and philosophy, he was a distinguished and successful practitioner of medicine and the author of many works highly prized for nearly five centuries, some of which are still reprinted.

He says pathetically, "Although from my youth Thorah was betrothed to me and continues to live by me as the wife of my youth, in whose love I find a constant delight, strange women, whom I took at first into my house as her handmaids, have become her rivals and absorbed part of my time." The spirit of the man is manifest in his famous prayer, one of the precious documents of our profession, worthy to be placed beside the Hippocratic oath. It ends with: "In suffering let me always see only my fellow creature."*

In the revival of learning in the thirteenth century, which led to the foundation of so many of the universities, Hebrew physicians took a prominent part, particularly in the great schools of Montpellier and of Paris, and for the next two or three centuries in Italy, in France and in Germany, Hebrew physicians were greatly prized. But too often the tribulations of Israel were their lot. As one reads of the grievous persecutions they suffered, there comes to mind the truth of Zunz' words: *"Wenn es eine Stufenleiter von Leiden giebt, so hat Israel die hochste Staffel erstiegen."* Their chequered career is well illustrated by the relations with the Popes, some of whom uttered official bulls and fulminations against them, others seem to have had a special fondness for them as body physicians. Paul III was for years in charge of Jacob Montino, a distinguished Jewish physician, who translated extensively from the Arabic and Hebrew into Latin, and his edition of Averroes is dedicated to Pope Leo X.

In my library there is a copy of the letter of Pope Gregory XIII, dated March 30th, 1581, and printed in 1584, confirming the decrees of Paul IV and Pius V, which he regrets were by no means held in observance, "but that there are still many among Christian persons who desiring the infirmities of their bodies to be cured by

*I am told by authorities that the attribution of this prayer to Maimonides is doubtful. Where is the original? W.O.

58

illicit means, and especially by the service of Jews and other infidels . . ." It was at Mantua that a Jewish physician, Abraham Conath, established a printing press, from which the first Hebrew works were issued. Throughout the sixteenth, seventeenth, and eighteenth centuries in France, Germany, and Italy we meet many distinguished names in the profession, and in his *Geschichte der Jüdischen Aertz,* Landau pays a very just tribute to their work. Only a few are met with in England. Isaac Abendana, a Spaniard, practised in Oxford and lectured on Hebrew at Magdalen College.

We have at the Bodleian, Jewish almanacs which he issued at the end of the seventeenth century, and a great Latin translation of the *Mischna.* He afterwards migrated to Cambridge. A more important author was Jacob de Castro Sarmento, a Portuguese Jew, who became licentiate of the Royal College of Physicians in 1725, and Fellow of the Royal Society in 1730. There is in the Bodleian an interesting broadsheet from the Register of the London Synagogues respecting charges made when his name was proposed at the Royal Society. He contributed many papers to the *Philosophical Transactions,* and was the author of several works.

In the eighteenth century Jean Baptiste de Silva, of a Portuguese Jewish family, became one of the leading physicians of Paris, consulting physician to Louis XV, and the friend of Voltaire, who remarks, *"C'ètait un de ces médecins que Molière n'eut ni pu ni osé rendre ridicules."* One of the special treasures of my library is a volume of the *Henriade* superbly bound by Padeloup, and a presentation copy from Voltaire to de Silva, given me when I left Baltimore by my messmates in The Ship of Fools.* Voltaire's inscription reads as follows:

"À Monsieur Silva, Esculape François. Recevez cet hommage de votre frère en Apollon. Ce Dieu vous a laissé son plus bel héritage, tous les Dons de l'esprit, tous ceux de la raison, et je n'eus que des Vers, hélas, pour mon partage."

In the nineteenth century, with the removal of the vexatious restrictions, the Jew had a chance of reaching his full development, and he has taken a position in the medical profession comparable to that occupied in the palmy Arabian days at Cordova and Baghdad. In Germany particularly, the last half of the century witnessed a remarkable outburst of scientific activity. Traube, who

*A dining club.

59

may well be called the father of experimental pathology; Henle, the distinguished anatomist and pathologist; Valentin, the physiologist; Lebert, Remak, Romberg, Ebstein, Henoch, have been among the clinical physicians of the very first rank. Cohnheim was the most brilliant pathologist of his day; to Weigert pathological histology owes an enormous debt, and, to crown all, the man whose ideas have revolutionized modern pathology, Paul Ehrlich, is a Jew.

In America Hebrew members of our profession for many years occupied a very prominent position. The father of the profession today, a man universally beloved, is Abraham Jacobi, full of years and honours; and the two most brilliant representatives in physiology and pathology, Simon Flexner and Jacques Loeb, carry out the splendid traditions of Traube and Henle.

I have always had a warm affection for my Jewish students, and it has been one of the special pleasures of my life the friendships I have made with them. Their success has always been a great gratification, as it has been the just reward of earnestness and tenacity of purpose and devotion to high ideals in science; and, I may add, a dedication of themselves as practitioners to everything that could promote the welfare of their patients. In the medical profession the Jews had a long and honourable record, and among no people is all that is best in our science and art more warmly appreciated; none in the community take more to heart the admonition of the son of Sirach—"Give place to the physician, let him not go from thee, for thou hast need of him."

xxv. *Looking Back—1889**

THAT those of us in control of departments at its opening should have been spared to see this twenty-fifth anniverary of the hospital is a piece of singular good fortune. It is a small matter that Iam not with you. "Where the greater malady is fixed, the lesser is scarce felt" expresses my feeling in the present crisis. You all know how I would have enjoyed the reunion with so many so dear to me by the strongest ties that bind man to man—the same ideals in life, the same pride in a splendid heritage, and that sense of close comradeship enjoyed by men who have initiated a great work and have survived to see it successful beyond their wildest dreams.

The Johns Hopkins Foundations were only grafts on the educational tree, grafts that would have withered had they not partaken of the root and fatness—to use a Biblical phrase—of its natural branches. Great biologists before Martin, great physicists before Rowland, great chemists before Remsen, great Grecians before Gildersleeve had had their day in America. It was not the men, though success could not have come without them, so much as the method, the organization, and a collective new outlook on old problems. They were gathered here from all parts to do one thing, to show that the primary function of a university was to contribute to the general sum of human knowledge. On the way they could teach and they had to teach what the fathers had taught, but this was only a means to a definite end, viz., in science and in arts to widen man's outlook so as to strengthen his dominion over the forces of nature.

Individuals here and there for generations had had in this country these ideals, but never before a *studium generale,* a whole body of men gathered in one place to form a university. That part of the university which, with the hospital, forms the medical school has only had twenty-five years of existence, not a generation, a mere fraction of time in the long history of the growth of science, so that it seems presumptuous to claim any powerful influence on the profession at large. The feeling, however, is strong, too strong to be passed over, that the year 1889 did mean something in the history

*Remarks read for Professor Osler at the Johns Hopkins Celebration, 1914.

of medicine in this country. One thing certainly it meant, as originally designed by that great leader, Daniel C. Gilman, that the ideals of the men on this side of Jones Falls were to be the same as those of the men in the laboratories of North Howard Street, that a type of medical school was to be created new to this country in which teacher and student alike should be in the fighting line. That is lesson number one of our first quarter-century, judged by which we stand or fall.

And lesson number two was the demonstration that the student of medicine has his place in the hospital as part of its machinery just as much as he has in the anatomical laboratory, and that to combine successfully in his education practise with science, the academic freedom of the university must be transplanted to the hospital. Again, it was not men, but a method, initiated in Holland, developed in Edinburgh, matured in London, and long struggled for here, but never attained until the Johns Hopkins Medical School was started.

And binding us all together there came as a sweet influence the spirit of the place; whence we knew not, but teacher and taught alike felt the presence and subtle domination. Comradeship, sympathy one with another, devotion to work, were its fruits, and its guidance drove from each heart hatred and malice and all uncharitableness.

Looking back, these are my impressions of the work of the Johns Hopkins Hospital.

But I must touch a personal note, and pay a tribute of affection to the men who helped to make my special clinic. In those early days of happy memories Booker and Harry Thomas in the dispensary sowed the good seed which has thriven so wonderfully in great new departments. Lafleur, Reese, Toulmin, Scott, Thayer, Hewetson, Simon, Hoch, Frank Smith and Barker helped to organize in those plastic first years our methods of work. No one feature contributed more to the development of the hospital than the presence in each department of a group of senior assistants. I look with a justifiable pride at the work of these men. In succession during my term, Lafleur, Thayer, Futcher, McCrae, Emerson controlled the work, and my indebtedness to them cannot be expressed in words. Always loyal and considerate, no chief ever had more devoted helpers. And we were singularly fortunate in our assistants, senior and junior. The list is too long to tell over. Many

62

came from outside schools, but the spirit of the place soon came upon them. Scattered far and wide now in important posts, they know how my heart follows their work, and how proud I am of their success. To have more than thirty of one's "boys" actively engaged in teaching is to draw a big prize in the lottery of life, with which for solid satisfaction there is nothing to compare.

But shadows flit across the picture—dark memories of the men whose leaves perished in the green. Jack Hewetson we all loved, I as a son, Thayer and Barker and Frank Smith as a brother. There was a light in his blue-grey eyes that kindled affection in all who knew him. Meredith Reese, the first to go, stricken also with tuberculosis, left us with scarred hearts. Livengood, whose mental outfit promised a career of special brilliancy, met a tragic death in the Bourgogne. Lazear, who went from the clinical laboratory to join Walter Reed, died a martyr's death in Cuba.

Oppenheimer and Ochsner, men of great merit, died on duty in the hospital. John Bruce MacCallum, in intellect "the bright particular" among our students, lived long enough to snatch something from dull oblivion. Al. Scott, whom we all loved dearly, had a successful career in Philadelphia before the call came. And only recently we have to mourn two of our best—Rupert Norton was one of the finer spirits, only touched to fine issues in a suitable environment, and that he found here in the latter years of his all-too-brief life; Otto Ramsay, who came to our clinic first, became one of the most successful teachers and practitioners in New England.

The Johns Hopkins Hospital illustrates the growth of an idea, represented by the founder, and the intelligent coöperation of different units. The foundation stones were laid by the adviser, John S. Billings, by Francis T. King, the president, and by the Board of Trustees. Under the wise guidance at first of President Gilman, then for long years of Dr. Hurd, the organization grew apace, and the hospital was made a fit habitation for patients by the work of Miss Isabel Hampton, Miss Rachel Bonner, and Mr. Emery. The medical staff has used the facilities thus afforded for the benefit of the public, in curing the sick, in studying the nature of disease, and in training men to do the same, with what measure of success we must leave to the judgement of posterity. To me at any rate there remains a precious memory of the years I spent in Baltimore, and an enduring pride that I should have been associated with the work of this hospital.

xxvi. *Nathan Smith*

READERS of my occasional essays will recall how frequently I have referred to Dr. Nathan Smith as one of the pioneers of clinical medicine in the United States. Many years ago his *Practical Essay on Typhous Fever,* New York, 1824, fell into my hands, and I have always praised it as a model of accurate clinical description. He recognized that the autumnal fever of the United States was "a disease *sui generis* arising from a specific cause, and that cause contagion."

At Baltimore I was not a little interested to find that the leading practitioner of the city and one of the trustees of he Johns Hopkins Hospital was Dr. Alan Smith, a grandson of Nathan Smith. To him and to his family I was indebted for many acts of great kindness. One evening at his house Mrs. Smith brought out a box of family documents, which I saw at once had a unique value. They told the story of Nathan Smith and his association with the profession in new England, and particularly with the founding of the medical schools of Dartmouth, Yale, Burlington and Bowdoin. I forget whether it was then or later that I urged Mrs. Smith to put this material together and tell the story of one of the great names in the history of the profession in the United States. This she has now done in a charming volume issued from the Yale Press,* with an introduction by Professor Welch.

I saw enough of the correspondence to appreciate how valuable the records were for the history of medicine for the period between 1780 and 1830. It is a splendid story, well told in the best possible way, largely in first-hand letters. As Dr. Welch remarks, we have here presented a splendid picture of Nathan Smith's life, "of his struggles and trials, of his indomitable courage and resourcefulness, of his marvelous capacity for work, of his professional and educational ideals and activities, and of his triumphs. We catch intimate glimpses of the active-minded lad upon the frontier, of

The Life and Letters of Nathan Smith, by Emily A. Smith, New Haven. 1914.

64

the student at home and abroad, getting, in spite of great difficulties, a good medical training, of the lover 'transported with joy and expectation,' of the devoted husband and father, solicitous for the education of his sons, of the busy physician and surgeon, 'bandied about from one part of the country to the other,' treating fevers, couching for cataract, cutting for stone, excising tumours, and embarrassed most of the time, as is the way of doctors, from failure or inability to collect his fees, small as they were, of the founder of medical schools and the professor, fiilling and filling well all the chairs in the medical curriculum—from all accounts a really great teacher, and withal deserving President Woolsey's characterization of him as 'the most delightful, unselfish and kind-hearted man I ever knew, and we children all loved him.' "

I remember how strongly I was impressed by the letters between Nathan Smith and George Cheyne Shattuck, of Boston, the father, grandfather, and great-grandfather of the Shattucks who have helped to make the profession of Boston famous during the nineteenth century. Smith's letters show the energy and perseverance with which he set about the establishment of the Dartmouth Medical School. He taught anatomy, surgery, chemistry, and the theory and practise of medicine. Mr. Abraham Flexner in his report on American medical education speaks of him in relation to Dartmouth as a man who "was its entire faculty, and a very complete faculty at that." The classes increased with rapidity, so that in 1809 there were one hundred students. One of the chief struggles was to get material for dissection, as in those days, "the cutting up of dead bodies was a grievous offence to the public." One of Dr. Smith's chemistry lectures brought out the following unique prayer from President Wheelock, who came to college chapel direct from chemical class-room:

"Oh, Lord! we thank Thee for the Oxygen gas; we thank Thee for the Hydrogen gas; and for all the gases. We thank Thee for the Cerebrum; we thank Thee for the Cerebellum, and for the Medulla Oblongata."

It is nice to know that Nathan Smith's name has been honoured at Dartmouth in connexion with the splendid new laboratory for chemistry and pathology.

Largely owing to Smith's untiring energy and ability as a practitioner and teacher, the reputation of the Dartmouth school increased with great rapidity, and it is not surprising that in 1813 he was called upon by Yale College to help in the establishment of a medical school at New Haven. Opening with thirty students the school grew rapidly under his fostering care. It is interesting to note that in connexion with it he early planned a botanical garden. It was not until 1817 that he severed his connexion finally with Dartmouth, and moved to New Haven. In 1821 he helped to found the Maine Medical College at Bowdoin, and lectured there for ten weeks in each year on anatomy, surgery and medicine, from 1821 to 1823. It was at this period that he did one of the notable operations in surgery, not knowing that it had been done before by McDowell—the successful removal of an ovarian cyst. In 1820, he helped his son, Nathan R., to organize the medical school at Burlington, Vermont. Nor did his energy in establishing schools end here, for his services were enlisted in the founding of the Jefferson Medical College, Philadelphia, in which his son, Nathan R., and Dr. George McClellan took a leading part. Early in 1829 he had a stroke, which fortunately carried him off without a long illness.

Nathan Smith was of the very best type of New England physician, of untiring energy, strong mental and moral qualities, and characterized above all by good plain common sense. His name deserves to be held in reverence, and I am sure this story of his life, so well told by the widow of his grandson, will be warmly appreciated by the profession.

UNITY, PEACE, AND CONCORD

A farewell address to the Medical Profession of the United States,
delivered before the Medical and
Chirurgical Faculty of the State of Maryland, 1905.

IT MAY be that in the hurry and bustle of a busy life I have given
offence to some—who can avoid it? Unwittingly I may have shot
an arrow o'er the house and hurt a brother—if so, I am sorry, and
I ask his pardon. So far as I can read my heart, I leave you in
charity with all. I have striven with none, not for the reason given
by Walter Savage Landor, because none was worth the strife, but
because I had a deep conviction of the blessings that come with
unity, peace, and concord. And I would give to each of you, my
brothers—you who hear me now, and to you who elsewhere may
read my words—to you who do our greatest work, labouring incessantly for small rewards in towns and country places—to you
the more favored ones who have special fields of work—to you
teachers and professors and scientific workers—to one and all,
through the length and breadth of the land—I give a single word
as my parting commandment:

> *It is not hidden from Thee, neither is it far off.*
> *It is not in heaven, that Thou shouldest say,*
> *"Who shall go up for us to heaven, and bring it unto us,*
> *that we may hear it, and do it?"*
> *Neither is it beyond the sea, that Thou shouldest say,*
> *"Who shall go over the sea for us, and bring it unto us,*
> *that we may hear it, and do it?"*
> *But the word is very high unto Thee, in Thy mouth,*
> *and in Thy heart, that Thou mayest do it*—CHARITY.

MEN AND BOOKS was first privately published in book form by Earl F. Nation, MD, in an edition of 250 copies printed by the Castle Press in 1959. The present edition is reprinted from one of those copies with Dr. Nation's kind permission.

Of this edition one thousand copies have been printed. The blue Fabriano paper of the binding recalls Osler's affiliation with Oxford, where the papers were written, and the red linen that with McGill University, to which they were sent.

G. S. T. Cavanagh